IRRITABLE
BOWEL
SYNDROME
AND
DIVERTICULOSIS

D0169497

For Whom is This Book Written?

Anyone who has been diagnosed by a doctor as having the Irritable Bowel Syndrome.

Do remember: *All persistent abdominal symptoms should be investigated, and only when you have been given this diagnosis and when the prescribed treatment fails to relieve the symptoms should self-help measures be used.*

Irritable Bowel Syndrome and Diverticulosis

A *Self-help plan*

Shirley Trickett

Thorsons

While the author of this work has made every effort to ensure that the information contained in this book is as accurate and up to date as possible at the time of publication, medical and pharmaceutical knowledge is constantly changing and the application of it to particular circumstances depends on many factors. Therefore it is recommended that readers always consult a qualified medical specialist for individual advice. This book should not be used as an alternative to seeking specialist medical advice, which should be sought before any action is taken. The author and publishers cannot be held responsible for any errors and omissions that may be found in the text, or any actions that may be taken by a reader as a result of any reliance on the information contained in the text, which is taken entirely at the reader's own risk.

Thorsons
An Imprint of HarperCollins*Publishers*
77–85 Fulham Palace Road,
Hammersmith, London W6 8JB

Illustrations by Peter Cox

First published by Thorsons 1990
This revised edition published 1999

10 9 8 7 6 5 4 3

A catalogue record for this book
is available from the British Library

ISBN 0 7225 3861 8

Printed and bound in Great Britain by
Creative Print and Design (Wales), Ebbw Vale

Contents

Part Two – Self-Help Methods

Part Three – Complementary Medicine

Foreword

This is an extremely well written and very comprehensive guide to self improvement and self help for people with bowel disorders. The scope of the book is so broad that anyone with even the most minimal tummy problems would find their health considerably improved by following some, if not all, of the advice given. Shirley Trickett has addressed almost every aspect of alternative and complementary medicine which may be able to offer help with these problems.

The problem of irritable bowel syndrome, or chronic constipation, diarrhoea, wind, bloating and associated anxiety, is one of the most common problems seen in medical practice. By addressing particularly the yeast overgrowth problem and food allergy, one is able to help the majority of sufferers, which is an idea that conventional medicine is currently slow to accept. Therefore, a book like this, designed to help the individual patient get on top of their own problem, is not only helpful for specific bowel problems, but it is also good for the person's self esteem to be able to approach their problem directly and feel that healing is within their own grasp.

It is, however, important to remember that most vitamins have associated toxicity problems and should not be taken indiscriminately, and a practitioner qualified in understanding vitamin medication should be consulted before a supplement programme is continued long term. I think it is also important to emphasize that diagnosis is critical. If your problems are wind, bloating, constipation, diarrhoea or mucus in your stools, it is important to first exclude that there is nothing else wrong with your bowel before assuming your problem is irritable bowel syndrome.

If used as a guide for self-improvement and restoration of general health, this book is likely to help many many sufferers from this disabling and crippling condition.

Dr Belinda Dawes B.M.B.S.

Preface

Half of all people whose bowel symptoms are investigated in hospital gastroenterology units are diagnosed as having the Irritable Bowel Syndrome. It can be a painful, debilitating condition and is second only to back pain as a cause of lost working hours. In view of this it is surprising that modern conventional medicine usually has so little to offer.

In the course of my work in the community over the past 15 years I have met an alarming number of people whose symptoms have been diagnosed as the Irritable Bowel Syndrome. This blanket diagnostic label seems to mean: 'The results of our investigations are negative; you do not have any serious disease – but we do not really know what is causing your symptoms.'

Is a High-Fibre Diet Really the Answer for Everyone?

Patients are urged to eat a high-fibre diet – bran with everything (a reliable short cut to becoming mineral deficient or compounding a wheat allergy); and some are given drugs to help the bowel muscles relax. The diet usually makes matters worse, and for many what they had previously experienced as discomfort becomes a much sharper pain after following this eating plan. A few find the drugs helpful but many do not like their side-effects, or else do not find the improvement significant enough to warrant their continued use.

A typical case would be the patient who is initially delighted when told there is nothing seriously wrong but gets progressively more unhappy as the symptoms persist. He or she returns again and again to a GP with a recalcitrant bowel which is not responding to the suggested treatment. The 'Thick File Syndrome' – usually reserved for anxious and depressed patients – then develops.

To be fair, some doctors admit they are perplexed by this condition and refer their patients to an immunologist, or a gastro-enterologist with an interest in food intolerance. Other doctors suggest a doctor who specializes in clinical nutrition; unfortunately there are few doctors in the National Health Service who have specialized in this subject, and private medicine is beyond the means of many people.

The work of the clinical nutritionists (formerly clinical ecologists) suggests there are many causes of the Irritable Bowel Syndrome and happily good results can be achieved by relatively simple measures, such as adjusting the diet or life-style, 'spring cleaning' the bowel, and encouraging the growth of helpful bacteria.

The Purpose of This Book

This is an optimistic book which aims to help you discover why your bowel is not functioning normally and how you can help it to heal. It could also explain some of your other apparently unrelated symptoms by showing how crucial a healthy bowel is to the health of the whole body. Troubles which seem remote from the abdomen, such as aching joints, depression, and headaches, can disappear as harmony is restored in the bowel. 'Spring cleaning' of the bowel is explained, as is how to protect it if you need to take prescribed drugs such as antibiotics, and several diets are suggested.

It is hoped that the information given here will help you to change the 28 feet of muscular tubing that you carry around in your abdomen from the equivalent of a main-drain system to a clean efficient factory where nutrients are absorbed and vitamins are manufactured. You will also be shown how to promote the growth of helpful bacteria – organisms which are ever-ready to stop other, wayward organisms like *Candida Albicans* causing chronic ill health by producing putrefaction and chemical mayhem in the bowel. Your part will be to feed the conveyor belt with clean, nutritious food and take an honest look at your general health.

It is also hoped that the following pages will help you to leave behind all those murmurings that have cruelly eroded your self-esteem at a time when you already felt ill and defeated. No doubt you will be familiar with some of these: 'Of course he is that certain personality type/Is she on about her bowel again?/You do realize you are causing these symptoms yourself don't you?/It's just stress' and so on. If you are willing to leave all this behind and accept you may have to make some major changes in your life, such as foregoing some of your favourite foods, doing tedious exercises, and making time for relaxation, you could restore your bowel to normal functioning and dramatically improve the quality of your life. Good health is just around the bend!

PART
ONE

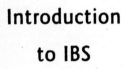

Introduction
to IBS

I

What is the Irritable Bowel Syndrome?

Irritable Bowel Syndrome (IBS) is the name given to a disorder of the muscular walls of the bowel. It affects gut motility – the rate at which the contents of the bowel are pushed along to the rectum – and is characterized by abdominal pain or discomfort, constipation, diarrhoea or alternate bouts of constipation and diarrhoea. These symptoms are common to most sufferers, but there are also a host of other symptoms associated with the condition; the nature of these depends on the cause of the problem. So, while several people could be diagnosed as having Irritable Bowel Syndrome, their symptoms could vary a great deal; for example, symptoms of IBS caused by milk intolerance could be very different from those symptoms where the problem is the result of stress or of an infection.

Irritable Bowel Syndrome is also known by other names: Mucous Colitis, Spastic Colon, or Non-inflammatory Bowel Disease. The term Irritable Bowel Syndrome seems to be a misnomer, for the bowel of the majority of sufferers – far from being irritable – is half-asleep. Since the treatment should vary according to exactly how the bowel is behaving, it would seem appropriate to give this condition three names: the Sluggish Bowel Syndrome, the Hyperactive Bowel Syndrome and the Confused Bowel Syndrome, the latter describing the alternate bouts of constipation and diarrhoea. These variations will be discussed fully later.

Who Suffers from this Condition?

Irritable Bowel Syndrome affects all age groups, from the infant who cries with colic to the aged. It ranges in degree from just a temporary interruption in an otherwise normal life, to a condition which makes a person look ill-nourished, constantly tired, miserable and confused.

What Are the Symptoms of Irritable Bowel Syndrome?

- *Abdominal pain, aching, heaviness*
- *excessive wind*
- *bloating*
- *constipation*
- *diarrhoea*
- *incontinence*
- *mucus in the stool*
- *small ribbon or pebble-like bowel movements*
- *rectal discomfort, never feeling the rectum is completely cleared*
- *poor appetite, weight loss*
- *wanting to eat frequently to 'move things along', weight gain*
- *tightness around the waist*
- *headaches, backache*
- *anxiety*
- *depression*
- *painful periods, painful intercourse*
- *difficulty bending down*

Other Symptoms Often Associated With Irritable Bowel Syndrome

- *Sore mouth, stinging tongue, swollen lips*
- *raw feeling in the gullet*
- *breathing problems*
- *restlessness*
- *difficulty getting to sleep, waking one hour after dropping off*
- *rapid pulse (or occasionally slow pulse)*
- *flushing after food*
- *fluid retention*
- *aching joints*
- *rashes*
- *fatigue*
- *cystitis which does not respond to antibiotics, frequent passing of urine without pain*
- *panic attack or depression after eating.*

The reasons for these odd symptoms will become clearer after the causes of Irritable Bowel Syndrome have been discussed.

Chapter 2 looks at some of the causes of persistent abdominal symptoms which defy routine investigations and do not respond to conventional treatment.

2

What Causes the Irritable Bowel Syndrome?

Anything which depresses the immune system, the body's defence against disease and foreign proteins, or anything which disturbs the balance of the gut flora allowing the 'bad' bacteria to take over can cause IBS. This could be:

When we are physically run down:
After infections, particularly bowel infections; after surgery; after childbirth; living with chronic physical pain; during hormonal upsets.

When we are emotionally low:
Coping with life situations such as illness, bereavement, overwork and relationship difficulties.

When we have an overgrowth of *Candida Albicans* (Thrush) in our gut:
Often characterized by craving for sweet foods.

When we have food allergies or intolerances:
These are becoming increasingly common and are often associated with *Candida*.

When prescribed drugs have affected the bowel:
It has been known for some time that antibiotics can upset the
bowel long term; other drugs are implicated too (page 92).

When we are lacking in essential nutrients:
For example some of the B vitamins are essential for the health of
the bowel.

When we are not producing enough digestive enzymes:
Why this happens is discussed in the problems of the toxic colon on
page 50.

When our blood sugar levels are unstable:
This can cause carbohydrate craving and lead to poor nutrition and
a toxic colon.

When we hyperventilate:
Overbreathing can lead to abdominal troubles through air-
swallowing and tension, and could possibly be a factor in allergies.

Why Are There so Many Sufferers?

The short answer is that living in the twentieth century has become
a health hazard. People who don't want to accept this often declare
we have become a society of malingerers or that the root causes of
Irritable Bowel Syndrome are all psychosomatic. It cannot be denied
that nervous tension is often part of the picture, but there are great
dangers in always focusing solely on this as a cause.

History has shown that non life-threatening illnesses are often
fashionable for a while then disappear; like the bustle or flared
trousers, the vapours and grumbling appendices came and went.
Unfortunately it seems unlikely that the Irritable Bowel Syndrome
will become outmoded until we listen to the cries of our over-
burdened immune systems and harken to the groaning of our gut.
We cannot expect our bodies to behave normally when they have to
cope with the pace of modern life, prescribed drug damage, antibiotics and hormones in meat, environmental pollution and careless
nutrition. The human body is a wonderful creation but even the
best biological systems have their breaking point.

Before the causes of Irritable Bowel Syndrome are looked at in more detail, and you discover what is causing your symptoms, it would be useful to look briefly at how the digestive system works and what the bowel needs to keep it healthy.

Understanding the Digestive System

The Mouth

Digestion starts in the mouth where food is chewed and mixed with saliva. This contains water salts and the enzyme ptyallin which breaks down starch. Mucus is also secreted in the mouth to lubricate the food. *If meals are swallowed hastily without being adequately chewed this important first stage of digestion is incomplete.*

The Gullet and Stomach

The food then passes down the gullet, or oesophagus, to the stomach where it is churned to break it up and mixed with gastric juices which break down the contents, kill germs and generally prepare it to enter the small intestine.

The Small Intestine

This is a coiled muscular tube about 20–24 feet in length. The functions of this tube are digestion and absorption. Very little food is

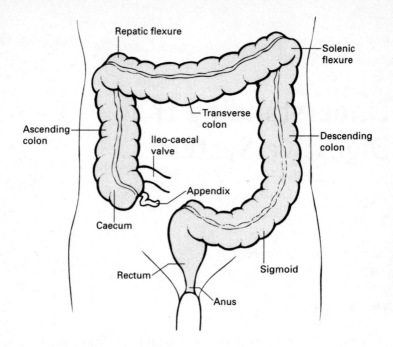

Fig 1. Normal colon

absorbed from the stomach; absorption takes place almost entirely from hair-like projections, called villi, on the wall of the intestines.

The Bowel

Food then travels to the bowel or colon – a wider tube about 5–6 feet long. By the time the material reaches here it contains very little food. The residue consists of water, salts, cellulose (the indigestible parts of fruit and vegetables) and bacteria. Although the stomach juices have killed off most of the germs, the ideal conditions of food and moisture enable the remaining ones to flourish. In the bowel, water and salts are quickly absorbed, leaving a paste called the stool or faeces. The few inches of tube which holds the stool before it is expelled is called the rectum. This is normally empty, but when it is full, the sensation produced brings the desire to empty the bowel.

This sensation frequently occurs when food or drink are taken, particularly the first hot drink in the morning. The first cigarette of the day also stimulates the bowel; people often become very constipated when they stop smoking.

Classifying the Irritable Bowel Syndrome

After reading the previous chapter it should be easier to understand where your symptoms are coming from. Is the stool delayed in the bowel, where it becomes too hard and dry to pass comfortably? Have the muscles given up trying? Or is the bowel so overstimulated that the stool rushes through before the fluid can be extracted, making the bowel movement watery and urgent?

In summary, do you have:

a   A *sluggish bowel*
b   A *hyperactive bowel*
c   A *confused bowel?*

Unless you have definite signs of *Candida* or food intolerance you can adjust your diet to either slow down or speed up the muscular action of the bowel. However, it would be pointless to do this without also gearing down and building relaxation into your day (see page 120). If your symptoms are not severe, you could try the following simple suggestions, before looking for problems such as allergies.

Trying the Common-Sense Approach

If your bowel is not functioning normally it is saying very clearly that it does not like the treatment it is receiving. It may be your diet, lack of exercise, loss of tone in the abdominal muscles, or your state of mind.

The Needs of the Sluggish Bowel

Start by drinking more water, particularly on waking and between meals. If you drink water with meals it dilutes the gastric juices which is not beneficial. Eat foods with a high water content, vegetables (particularly raw), and fruit. A high-fibre diet does not need to be a high-bran diet. It is better if whole grains are eaten instead of adding extra bran, as extra bran can sometimes lead to irritation of the lining of the bowel or prevent the absorption of some minerals.

Take a Bulking Agent

This is a substance which soothes the lining of the bowel and surrounds the hard pellets of faeces, making a spongy mass which stimulates peristalsis, the wavelike muscular contraction of the wall of the bowel. *Psyllium* or *Ispagula* husk, from a plant in the plantain family, is an excellent choice and is available in most pharmacies and health food stores. It is old-fashioned, cheap and less likely to cause irritation or allergy than bran-based products. Isogel is one brand, but there are others. (New Nutrition have a range of colon cleansing products: see page 210).

How do I Take it?

The dose is 1–2 teaspoonfuls in water daily. It has little taste and is not a problem to take, although mixing it with carbonated water does make it easier to get down. It must be swallowed immediately after mixing; you will see by the remains in the glass that it quickly forms a jelly. Linseed is also soothing and healing for the bowel, and most health food shops and some pharmacies have it. If you soak a few seeds in water you will see a jelly form. This has the same action as the Isogel and in addition has nutritional benefits. One dessertspoonful can be taken in yogurt or on cereal in the mornings, or you can keep a bowl on the table and take a few every time you pass, making sure you chew them thoroughly because they are a good source of essential fatty acids. A product called Linuset Gold can be found in most health food shops.

Avoid Laxatives

These only store up more trouble because you cannot re-educate your bowel by continually giving it stimulants such as phenolphthalein, senna or bisacodyl. If you have to take anything take something which has nutritional benefits, such as vitamin C or magnesium.

Vitamin C is necessary for the health of the bowel and is a great boost for the immune system. If you are very constipated the dose will be above 2 gm daily; a useful way to find out how much to take is to gradually increase the dosage until you get diarrhoea, then reduce it until the stool is formed and comfortable. Many alternative medical practitioners believe you will not get diarrhoea until your body has selected the dose it needs. If this is so the person who smokes and has a poor diet should be able to take several grams before diarrhoea results. Permanent improvement, of course, must come from diet and your way of life.

CAUTION

Vitamin C, as has been said, can cause abdominal discomfort and diarrhoea and can also, for some people, be very stimulating. Take it in the mornings to avoid insomnia. If you are a very nervous person start with a low dose – say 25 mg – and increase gradually. Vitamin C is vital for the immune and nervous systems. If you cannot take supplements make sure you get plenty of fresh fruit and vegetables. Shortage of vitamin C is associated with an increase in allergic reactions.

The Sluggish Bowel Needs Exercise

Consider what you are doing with your body all day long; how you are restricting your abdominal muscles by the way you sit, by tight clothing or permanent tension. Walking or cycling to work, swimming or just doing a few simple stretch exercises every day can prevent constipation. More about this later.

Why it is So Painful

It is strange that the bowel can be cut without pain; it is the stretching of the wall beyond its normal limits that causes such agony. When the bowel is blocked with hard faeces wind cannot be expelled and the pressure builds up. If you are very uncomfortable you could use an occasional laxative or two glycerine suppositories, which you will find in any pharmacy. These cone-shaped jellies, about an inch long, draw water from the rectal wall, soften the stool and stimulate the desire to move the bowel. The best position for insertion is to lie on your side with your knees drawn up to the chest. If you moisten the pointed end of the suppository in warm water it should be quite pain-less to insert it high into the rectum; your finger should be protected by a rubber finger-cot (a protective covering rather like the finger of a rubber glove) or a double layer of clingfilm. It will be easier to retain the suppositories longer if you stay lying down and do some slow breathing. You might have the desire to move your bowel after a few minutes, but try to hang on; if you can manage ten to fifteen minutes you should have a more satisfactory result.

Some people buy enema kits from surgical stores or order them by mail order through health magazines, and find a warm water enema very helpful. Perhaps it would be better to ask your doctor before you take this step.

Can the Doctor Give Me Anything for the Pain?

Yes. This would either be something for the constipation such as Bisacodyl tablets or Picolax powder, or something to relieve the spasm in the smooth muscle of the bowel such as Merbentyl (dicylomine hydrochloride), Colofac (mebeverine hydrochloride), or peppermint oil in capsules called Colpermin.

Is There Anything I Can Buy from the Pharmacists?

Dicycolome hydrochloride comes in a mixture called Kolanticon which is on free sale. You can also buy Colpermin capsules but they are rather expensive. The health food shop will also have peppermint preparations.

What Are the Drawbacks of Taking Drugs?

Any drug you take for the bowel should be regarded as a temporary measure to gain relief while you are treating the cause of the problem. The dangers of taking laxatives long-term have been discussed. Merbentyl and Colofac may cause dry mouth with difficulty swallowing, palpitations and flushing, constipation, difficulty passing water and slight confusion. Kolanticon could have the same effects and could also be unsuitable for people who are sensitive to aluminium. Peppermint preparations can cause heartburn and slight discomfort in the bladder and rectum. If there is any inflammation in the bowel it is unlikely that peppermint would be tolerated.

A Healthy Bowel Movement

This should be bulky, soft and mid-brown in colour; it should smell very little and disintegrate easily in the water of the lavatory.

A Constipated Bowel Movement

Because it has lost more water it is dark and compacted; it can also be streaked with mucus or blood. Blood in the stool must always be investigated even if you feel it is the result of straining to pass the hard faeces. Sometimes this opens up a crack (fissure) around the anus or causes a pile (haemorrhoid) to bleed.

Haemorrhoids

These varicose veins of the rectum are often the butt of music hall jokes, but any sufferer will tell you there is not a lot to laugh about; it is a very painful condition. Local anaesthetic creams and suppositories are on free sale at the pharmacy or can be prescribed by your doctor. They can make life a lot more bearable, but you cannot be really comfortable until you are no longer passing a hard stool. Your doctor will decide whether any medical treatment such as tying off the veins is necessary. The old remedy for piles was to scrape a clove of garlic to release the juice and then put it in the rectum. The effect is probably similar to eating a crushed clove; a fierce heat followed by a soothing warmth.

Causes of Constipation

Causes of constipation include:

- *Lack of water*
- *lack of fibre*
- *disturbance of the balance of the gut bacteria*
- *tension in the muscles of the colon, rectum and anus*
- *eating too much concentrated protein (eggs, cheese)*
- *the effects of some drugs; for example, iron tablets, codeine, tranquillizers, sleeping pills, anti-depressants, beta-blockers, water pills, some anti-histamines, Tagamet and Zantac (for stomach ulcers), some antacid preparations, some anti-convulsant drugs*
- *putting off going to the lavatory when you have had the signal to go*
- *pelvic congestion due to lax muscles or pre-menstrual tension.*

When the Bad Bacteria Take Over

In a healthy bowel three to four pounds of bacteria (the gut flora) work away to complete digestion, make vitamins and kill off bad bacteria, viruses, fungi and parasites, thus keeping the contents of the gut 'sweet'. If the bad bacteria take over the stool becomes 'sour' from putrefaction and a great deal of gas is formed. This is where the bloating and discomfort comes from.

Wind – Mounting Pressure

It is not only trying to pass a hard motion that causes pain; a colicky pain can be experienced when the bowel is trying to move the hard faeces through the colon, or when wind which cannot escape causes the bowel to stretch to a point where it contracts in protest and causes a sharp pain.

In a Yorkshire churchyard apparently there is a headstone which offers words of wisdom on this subject:

Wherever ye be let the wind go free
For stoppage of it was the death of me

Sound advice, but not always possible when you are constipated.

Fighting the Flatulence

Mild Symptoms

You could try fennel or peppermint tea, an adult dose of baby's gripe-water, half a teaspoonful or bicarbonate of soda in a glass of warm water, or a quarter of a teaspoonful of ginger in warm water. Fennel or caraway seeds after meals can help prevent wind; chew them very well. Charcoal biscuits, available from most pharmacies, are an old-fashioned remedy for wind. Sometimes eating a food such as garlic, onions, leeks or lentils which makes more wind and great rumblings (the strange medical name for noises in the gut is *borborygmi*) can serve to break up the stubborn wind and get things moving.

More Severe Symptoms

If you are quite sure that your trouble is no more than wind, a warm water enema or two glycerine suppositories can often bring immediate relief. Other measures include placing a covered hot water bottle on your abdomen as you lie on your back with your knees bent and feet flat on the floor, or getting into a warm bed with a compress made from a couple of cotton tea towels which have been soaked in very hot water. Squeeze out excess water, test the temperature carefully on your arm, then hold the compress in place with a large towel and get into bed. If you steam away nicely and relax, stay there and if possible have a nap; if you feel chilled get up and move around. Try it another time.

Massage

External

Massage with oil (olive is good) from the right groin up and above the navel then down the left side; continue for ten minutes. This also helps to break down and eliminate toxins. Another way is to rub the abdomen with the lightest possible touch in a clockwise circle; there is no need to undress. It is surprising how much gas is released from the stomach with this simple exercise.

Internal

Laughing is a good internal massage, but if you are full of wind your sense of humour will probably have deserted you. Controlled abdominal breathing is also helpful.

The Magic of Using Castor Oil Externally

When most people think of castor oil they imagine the horrors of swallowing it. There is no need for this. This old-fashioned remedy is extremely effective when applied to the skin.

For Constipation and Easing Bowel Discomfort

Castor oil is available in all pharmacies, usually in 3-oz bottles. The cold-pressed oil is best. You might be able to get this from a nutritionist or some health food stores.

CONSTIPATION:

1   Cut a piece of an old woollen vest, flannel, old blanket, lint, or any undyed absorbent material big enough to cover your abdomen.
2   Put it in a bowl or bathroom basin and soak thoroughly in the oil.
3   Massage the oil into the lower back and abdomen.
4   Wrap a hot water bottle (don't make it too hot to leave comfortably on the abdomen) in a wet tea towel or piece of old sheeting to make a steamy heat. Place this on the abdomen, making sure part of it is over the liver (under the ribs on the right side).
5   Get into a warm bed. Lie on a large towel and wrap the ends over you to protect the sheets.
6   Lie here for 30 minutes.
7   When you get up take a warm shower or bath.

If you put the oil-soaked cloth into a plastic bag it can be used up to three times before discarding or washing. You will of course need to add more oil. Since this simple treatment detoxifies the liver you might experience a slight dull ache in the liver area, which passes off usually within the hour. The oil goes through the skin to the internal organs, so don't be surprised if the stool has a strange odour or seems oily. You can do this daily until you get satisfactory results and then continue twice weekly or when you feel you need it.

WHOLE-BODY TREATMENT

This is wonderfully relaxing, detoxifying, helps constipation and can bring great relief to aching joints and muscles.

1   In a warm room, massage 3 oz of warm castor oil into the whole body starting on the neck, at the base of the skull. Pay particular attention to any painful area and the abdomen, base of the spine and feet. Cover these with white or pale-coloured cotton or woollen socks as soon as you have oiled them to prevent skidding on the bathroom floor.
2   Put on a pair of warmed light-coloured pyjamas or an old tracksuit, or wrap yourself in a warmed old sheet or large towel.

3 Get into a warmed bed (prepared before starting) and stay there overnight if possible.
4 Take a warm shower or bath when you get up, taking care to remove the oil from the soles of your feet before you step into the bath, to prevent slipping. You will find that a great deal of the oil has been absorbed during the night and, after washing, your skin will feel wonderfully soft.

CASTOR OIL BATH

This has the same benefits as the whole-body treatment but can be even more effective for painful joints and muscles.

1 Put soap, a sponge and two towels (one an old towel) near the bath, on a chair.
2 Run a comfortably warm bath and mix in a 3-oz bottle of castor oil.
3 Get in the bath, making sure the water is up to your neck and that the oil is dispersed. Lie there for 30 minutes.
4 Using the fresh towel at the edge of the bath, wash your hands and feet free of oil before you attempt to stand. Take great care because the bath will be very slippery. Use a bath mat and do not attempt to stand up until you have drained the bath, washed and dried it. You can then add clean water to remove oil from your body or you can take a shower.
5 If you are going to bed you can just towel-dry leaving a slight film of oil on. This should not feel sticky. If you use soap or shower gel, the oil can be completely removed.
6 If it is not bedtime, have a rest for at least half an hour in a warm bed or by the fire.

Using the Breath

If possible lie on the floor with your knees up and your feet flat on the floor; if this is not possible sit in a straight-backed chair and drop your shoulders. Breathe in and push your abdomen out; breathe out and pull your abdomen in and upwards towards the ribs. Continue for ten minutes. It would be surprising if this did not ease the spasm and allow you to get rid of some of the wind.

Pressure Points for Wind

Many alternative therapies share the belief (although they may have different names for it) that the body runs on a subtle form of electrical energy which runs in channels through the body. When the flow is interrupted in these channels – often by tension – discomfort or disease can result. Although there are many ways of correcting the energy flow, acupressure is one of the simplest. Here are some points to try.

1   *Let your arms hang by your sides and poke around on the outer edge of the thigh where your middle finger ends until you find a tender area; sometimes it feels as if you are pressing on grains of sand. Press or massage until you feel rumblings in your gut.*
2   *Hold out your arm and stick up your thumb as though you are hitching a lift. With the other hand feel around in the little depression right on the tip of the shoulder. Repeat for the other side. There can be some marked differences in these two points; if one side is very sore note what you do with that shoulder, are you holding it somewhere up around your ear? Tense shoulders play havoc with the digestive system.*

Homoeopathy for Wind

The science of homoeopathy has been practised in England since the 1850s, and because of disenchantment with highly technological medicine, more and more people are turning to it. Homoeopathy has been well-researched and has proven to be effective, not only in curing illness but also in preventing it. It uses only natural substances which are non-addictive and cheap. While it is better to go to a well-qualified homoeopathic practitioner, if this is not possible a considerable amount of relief can often be gained from reading simple first-aid homoeopathy instructions (see page 181) and buying the remedies from your chemist or health food shop.

Tissue Salts

Some people have also found *New Era Tissue Salts* very helpful.
These are easier to use than homoeopathic remedies because the
symptoms they are formulated to soothe are printed on the packages.
These salts are made into small moulded tablets and are also
homoeopathically prepared. They are very safe but may not be
suitable for people with severe milk intolerance because they
contain milk sugar.

Dr Bach Floral Remedies

Therapists and lay people alike are discovering how helpful these
flower and plant extracts are. They too are available, together with
an explanatory booklet, in health food shops. *Rescue Remedy*, a
mixture of extracts from five plants, is very popular and it is
surprising to see how many people carry it around in their brief
cases and handbags. Four drops on the tongue or in water for shock,
tension, exam nerves or general restlessness, can work wonders. It
also calms the digestive system.

The Overactive Bowel

You and your bowel need rest. Diarrhoea is usually the bowel's way
of getting rid of a substance it considers poisonous or is an
indication that your nervous system is worn out. If you are tense,
your muscles will be pumping out too much adrenalin and as a
result of this all your bodily functions, including the muscular action
of the bowel, will be speeded up. It may only be apparent in your
bowel but other parts could be affected too; breathing and heart rate
will increase, your muscles could feel restless and unable to relax,
your thoughts and speech could be more pressured. If your bowel is
reacting to stress, diet alone will not help; you will have to gear
down and make relaxation sessions as much a part of your day as
brushing your teeth. (Nervous diarrhoea is discussed on page 64.)

Resting the Bowel

If your stool is frequent and fluid, rest and take fluids only, but avoid milk and citrus drinks. Filtered, bottled or boiled water, apple juice or clear vegetable stock thickened with arrowroot or slippery elm powder (the pure powder, not the milk drink containing slippery elm), will both soothe and heal the bowel. White rice cooked in a lot of water until it becomes a creamy liquid has the same effect.

Taking a Bulking Agent for Diarrhoea

Isogel (or linseed) is as helpful for diarrhoea as it is for constipation. Take it with only enough fluid to get it down and it will act as a sponge and absorb excess fluid in the bowel.

Can my Doctor Give Me Anything for Diarrhoea?

Yes. It could be Imodium capsules (also available over the counter as Arret) or a kaolin and morphine mixture. Resort to medicine only when you have tried resting and fluids. There are two reasons for this. One is 'letting your guts have their say'; if they are trying to clean out toxins it is a mistake to interrupt this. The other reason is that although the drugs are certainly effective in stopping the diarrhoea, they can also leave you with constipation, and so the cycle goes on.

Coping with the Confused Bowel

If you have the type of IBS characterized by alternate bouts of constipation and diarrhoea, it is really the constipation that needs attention, because without this the diarrhoea would not develop. The lining of a dirty, constipated colon, can be so irritated by the toxins produced that it attempts to wash it away with a watery stool. Cleaning the bowel (page 52) and finding the correct diet are the answer if you are feeling the effects of the Toxic Colon Syndrome. Food allergy, *Candida*, or being over-anxious can also cause chronic diarrhoea.

5

If Your Colon is Inflamed

If the lining of the bowel is inflamed and swollen you could experience a lot of discomfort, and mucus or blood in the stool. *Your doctor must always investigate this.* Swelling in the lumen of the bowel often produces a flat, ribbon-like stool, which although it is soft can be difficult to pass. Old faeces can cling to the wall of the bowel and cause infection or inflammation. If your bowel is inflamed you will need to gently loosen this material, heal the lining and restore the balance of the gut flora by giving up junk foods and taking supplements. An inflamed bowel should not be attacked by laxatives or taking bran.

Gentle Cleansers

Psyllium husks or powder (available in health food stores or pharmacies) and slippery elm bark (a brown powder available from some health food stores and all nutritionists), taken with plenty of water, are gentle cleansers. When you start the psyllium you might find it gives you more wind, so start with half a teaspoonful and then graduate to the suggested dosage on the package – or follow the advice of your nutritionist. This supplement works well but you have to be patient. It could be several days before you are easily passing a soft but formed bulky stool. If your stool is very loose take this supplement with as little water as possible. You should not have any troubles with the slippery elm. It has a soothing effect on the whole of the digestive system and, incidentally, is also beneficial for the heart. One teaspoonful three times daily can be taken until symptoms improve.

Cleansing the bowel and healing with supplements need not go on for ever. When your symptoms improve you can gradually phase them out and use them intermittently when you feel you need them. In addition to the above you will need to avoid stress, keep to a healthy diet, drink plenty of water and take daily exercise (particularly walking) as much as possible. If you are elderly and cannot move about much, abdominal breathing and simple stretching exercises sitting in a chair will help.

Healing Supplements

L-Glutamine

It is only in the last 10 years that we have found that Glutamine is:

1   The primary nutrient for the digestive lining.
2   The primary fuel for the immune system.
3   Vital for the metabolism of muscle.
4   Vital for wound-healing and tissue repair.
5   The body's most common amino acid.

                                        Dr Douglas Wilmore, MD, Harvard Medical School

L-Glutamine is an amino acid used by nature to build proteins in the body. One of 20, it was formerly thought to be non-essential as it was thought it could be manufactured from other amino acids.

Glutamine in the diet comes from meat, fish and eggs, but cooking easily destroys it. There is barely enough glutamine in the diet if we are healthy. Extra glutamine may be needed during times of stress or after illness, infections or surgery.

Glutamine is the most popular anti-ulcer drug in Asia and its success in treating IBS and inflammatory bowel disease is remarkable. The range of illnesses (including mental illness) where L-Glutamine is proving to be invaluable is too wide to be discussed here. If you would like more information on this send to Higher Nature for Offprint 22, 'Glutamine Breakthroughs for Immunity, Muscle Strength and Healing the Digestive System' by Simon Martin (price at the time of writing is 30 pence).

This supplement is available through all nutritional suppliers in powder or capsule form. It is easier to take adequate doses in the powder form. It is white, tasteless and is taken just stirred into water.

Glucosamine (N-Acetyl-Glucosamine or NAG)

This is another very exciting supplement. Clinical studies are showing its value in a wide variety of conditions (for more information write to Higher Nature). Glucosamine is an amino sugar normally formed in the human body from glucose. It works well on its own or with L-Glutamine for many digestive problems including IBS, Colitis and Crohn's disease. It repairs and protects the lining of the digestive and urinary tract and enables nutrients to be more easily absorbed. Available from nutritionists and some health food stores.

The Aloe Vera Barbadensis Plant

The juice of this ancient, fleshy plant is the most versatile natural remedy known to modern science. It has 200 constituents including essential vitamins, minerals, proteins, lipids, 8 of the 10 amino acids necessary for health, and the unique aloe vera polysaccharides found only in this plant. Dr Ivan Danhof, MD, is universally acknowledged as the leading authority on the medicinal value of this plant. He is an eminent gastroenterologist and holds a professorship in biology and physiology. He is an independent consultant to a firm called Pro-Ma Systems who produce a high-quality aloe vera juice. This is not available in health stores. It is worth paying a little more for a good-quality, pure product.

For written information send SAE to:
Aloe Vera Centre (UK North)
Park Parade Therapy Clinic
58 Park Parade
Whitley Bay
Newcastle NE26 1DX
Or call/fax (0191) 252 4834 – Staff will be able to answer your
queries.

General Benefits of Aloe Vera Juice

- *helps arthritis*
- *lowers blood pressure and strengthens heart beat*
- *lowers cholesterol*
- *improves liver function*
- *increases skin and bone healing*
- *calms and heals the digestive tract*
- *balances blood sugar levels in diabetes or hypoglycaemia*
- *helps the immune system*

The list of conditions where aloe vera juice is helpful might seem
rather long and diverse, but when it is considered that the extract of
this plant is detoxifying, anti-inflammatory, anti-bacterial, antifungal,
is high in vitamins, minerals, amino acids and essential fatty acids, it
is not surprising that its applications are so wide.

Aloe Vera and IBS

Organic compounds in this juice can all be broken down to form
salicylates. These are both analgesic and anti-inflammatory and
inhibit the production of inflammatory prostaglandins from
arachiodonic acid.

The effect of faulty digestion in the stomach is discussed on page
32 in relation to IBS. Aloe vera can help to balance stomach acids,
assist in the breaking down of protein and therefore prevent
undigested molecules causing problems in the gut (see page 34).

The range of fatty acids produced by the plant includes linoleic,
mynistic, caprylic, oleic, palmitic and steraric acid – some of which

may not only be of value in lowering cholesterol but are also helpful in the production of useful prostaglandins which have anti-inflammatory properties.

Aloe vera has been found to have the anti-inflammatory action of steroid drugs like indomethacin and prednialone (for more information on this the Aloe Vera Centre – see above address).

Aloe Vera and Constipation or Diarrhoea

Research has shown aloe vera juice to be an adaptogen – that is, a substance capable of reducing diarrhoea if that is the problem, or in the case of constipation increasing bowel movements.

Will Aloe Vera Juice Help Abdominal Discomfort?

Yes, it will. There are several reasons why this is so:

1 *Improved digestion in the stomach, therefore less putrefaction – less gas*
2 *Food enters the bowel in a more acceptable state (protein molecules broken down – less gas)*
3 *Prevents overgrowth of bad bacteria and fungus such as candida albicans. Gas puts pressure on the gut wall. Ballooning or stretching of this wall causes pain.*
4 *Soothes and heals inflamed lining of bowel.*
5 *Inactivates a potent pain-producing agent and vasodilator (making blood vessels swell) called bradykinin.*

Food Intolerance and Aloe Vera

The juice can be helpful in several ways, including:

1 *The prevention of large molecules of undigested protein entering the bloodstream.*
2 *Vitamins and minerals are readily absorbed and some may be helpful in lowering allergic levels of histamine in the bloodstream.*
3 *Reduces inflammation caused by intolerances.*

IBS, Aloe Vera and the Skin

It is not surprising that digestive problems, joint and skin problems often go together. Many people find that when they have cleansed, healed and repopulated the digestive tract with good bacteria and also keep to a healthy diet, many long-term skin and joint conditions improve or disappear. These include arthritis, acne, acne roseacea, eczema, psoriasis, fungal skin problems, allergic skin troubles and many unnamed rashes. This makes sense. The toxins from the bowel often end up somewhere else. As has been said, the bowel should be a sealed unit but the 'leaky gut' syndrome is all too common.

Topical Use of Aloe Vera

Application of aloe vera to the skin is also very effective (but this does not mean that you can skip treating the bowel). Top-quality face and body preparations made to Dr Danhof's specifications are available from the Aloe Vera Centre – address above.

Essential Fatty Acids

These substances are vital for the health of the skin, immune and nervous systems. The modern diet is often deficient in them. The main sources are fatty fish, seeds: sunflower, sesame, pumpkin, linseed and starflower (borage), and oils from these seeds. Olive oil and Evening Primrose oils are also good sources. Signs of deficiency can be dry skin, inflammation in the digestive or urinary tract (sometimes a cause of microscopic blood in the urine – although this must never be taken as such and must be investigated by a doctor), and tingling in the limbs.

To be healthy a combination of Omega fatty acids 3, 6 and 9 are needed. Linseed (flax) taken with starflower should give all three. The linseed can be ground or soaked in water for better absorption (a jelly will form around the seeds). Flax oil is available from most health food stores and all nutritionists.

People often worry that taking oils will increase their weight. In fact the reverse of this can be true. Flax oil helps to rid the body of unwanted fluid. Evening Primrose oil can also help with excess weight by balancing hormone levels.

A supplement which contains all three oils is Essential Balance, available from New Nutrition and Higher Nature.

6

The Stomach and IBS

All digestive problems should be investigated by your doctor. If your doctor has found nothing wrong with your stomach and has given you antacids, if you don't respond to these it might be up to you to consider some other causes of poor digestion in the stomach.

Nervous Stomach

Worrying over anything can have a very bad effect on the stomach, but worrying over what you are actually eating can cause a great deal of problems – at the time when the digestive juices should be flowing you are stopping this natural process by negative thoughts – 'Can I eat this?/Dare I eat that?/Will I suffer after this?' and so on. The pleasure from eating is replaced by anxiety over what can be digested without discomfort, and so more and more foods are refused which further affects the nervous system and the immune system, already compromised by poor nutrition. People often see refined carbohydrates as foods that are easier to digest. If the diet is lacking in protein and roughage it might take quite a lot of refined carbohydrate to satisfy the appetite, with the result that a person with poor digestion can become both overweight and undernourished.

If on the other hand the appetite is poor, the 'Tea and Toast Syndrome' can develop.

It goes without saying that if tension and worry are affecting your digestive system, relaxing more will improve matters. Here is the experience of a young woman who in her own words became a 'food phobic'.

My life had been a nightmare for two years before I admitted it was simply stress and my own reactions to food that were causing my digestive problems. It started (although I only realize this now) when I was promoted at work. I was very keen to show my worth in the new position and often worked late or during my lunch break. I started to feel discomfort after my evening meal and always blamed what I had eaten. The range of foods I thought I could cope with dwindled. I lost weight and all pleasure from cooking and eating disappeared. I dreaded invitations to eat out. It was very embarrassing just picking at the food on my plate.

Last summer I went for an organized walking holiday in Wales. I was very nervous about my digestive problems, not only because I had to eat with 20 strangers but because I was also having difficulty getting off to sleep. It proved to be one of the best holidays I have had and gave me total insight into how I had become so neurotic about what I could and could not eat. I worried about food and did not sleep for the first couple of days, and then I think the fresh air and exercise must have taken over. I slept like a log and was hungry for the first time for months. I ate everything that was put in front of me without any discomfort at all.

My stomach still complains occasionally but I'm no longer fearful about this and can always see it is because I am trying to do too much.

Lack of Enzymes

When food enters the stomach it needs enzymes to help to break it down. If there is a deficiency of these substances then the small intestine has to cope with food which has not passed through the initial stages of digestion. The result is discomfort from wind and bloating. Taking supplements of digestive enzymes or eating a small amount of *well-chewed* raw vegetables before a cooked meal can help this problem – (see *Raw Energy* – in the Further Reading list). The pineapple is a good source of digestive enzymes. A piece of well-chewed pineapple or a glass of juice 10 minutes before eating can be helpful. Enzymes from the pineapple are also available in capsule form from nutritional suppliers.

Too Much Hydrochloric Acid

'Heartburn' or 'acid stomach' is an indication that you are producing too much hydrochloric acid because of the nervous state you are in. If you experience burning discomfort which is relieved by eating or if you regurgitate acid you could well be producing too much acid. Relieving these symptoms with antacids is fine as a first-aid measure but only in the short term.

If you are tense, the acid/alkaline balance in your stomach can be disturbed. You can make this worse by skipping or rushing meals, or by not eating enough alkaline-forming foods (see *Food Combining for Health* in the Further Reading list).

Water is a good and simple antacid. Drink plenty *between* meals.

Going to the Doctor with 'Acid Stomach' Problems

You might be given a simple antacid or a drug in the cimetidine group such as Tagamet. It cannot be denied that these drugs are effective – *but it is unwise to stay on them for long periods.*

Side-effects

I first came across large numbers of people who were given these drugs for gastro-intestinal disturbances when they were withdrawing from drugs in the benzodiazepine group such as diazepam or lorazepam. They were also given to people who were having withdrawal symptoms from antidepressant drugs such as amytriptyline or the MAOI inhibitors. (See *Coming Off Tranquillizers, Sleeping Pills and Antidepressants* in the Further Reading list.)

Many were left on cimetidine on repeat prescription for long periods without review. Long after the tranquillizer or antidepressant withdrawal was over many people reported feeling ill when they tried to stop cimetidine. A rebound over-production of gastric acid could be expected, but they also reported: irritability, insomnia, panic attacks and feeling generally very low. On the positive side, many users said that the bowel symptoms such as constipation and colic (many had suffered this for years) disappeared within two weeks of the discontinuation of the cimetidine or allied drug.

Fungal infections of the skin and gastro-intestinal tract have also been reported with these drugs ('Invasive Candidiasis Following Cimetidine Therapy', *American Journal of Gastroenterology*, 1, January 1983, pages 102–3).

My book *Coping with Candida – Are Yeast Infections Draining Your Energy?* (published by Sheldon Press) covers all aspects of fungal infections.

Cimetidine (Tagamet – a weaker version of the prescription drug) is now on free-sale in the UK. If it helps, use only in the short term (and not before you have had a firm diagnosis from your doctor). If it make you feel anxious or irritable you would be well advised to look for a natural approach to the problem of overacidity, such as changing your diet and lifestyle. If the symptoms persist, see your doctor with a view to some investigations. If your doctor is unwilling to see if you are producing too much or too little hydrochloric acid, this test can be arranged by a doctor who practises Clinical Nutrition (See British Society for Nutritional Medicine in the Useful Addresses chapter – you might need a referral from your GP).

Too Little Hydrochloric Acid

The body is always striving for balance; therefore it is not surprising that stress can also result in an underproduction of hydrochloric acid. It is very confusing because the symptoms can be similar to overproduction of acid and people often compound these symptoms by taking antacids.

Symptoms include excessive burping, a feeling of fullness after even a moderate meal, bad breath (which comes from food fermenting in the stomach). If the symptoms are severe, nausea, vomiting, bloating, wind and diarrhoea or constipation can result.

The presence of undigested food in the stool often indicates that food is not being digested in the stomach. Proteins (meat, fish, eggs, dairy produce, pulses) are the most difficult to digest. Large undigested protein molecules in the intestines can damage the lining and lead to food intolerances, allergies, overgrowth of 'bad' organisms and inflammation.

The production of hydrochloric acid declines with age, and even if a good diet is taken if it reaches the bowel in a half-digested state, then vital minerals and vitamins may not be absorbed. Eating when you are tired, bolting food or over-eating all make hard work for the stomach, and in the case of the latter a small amount of acid has to go a long way.

How Do I Know If I Am Over- or Underproducing Acid?

If your symptoms do not respond to antacids or changing your lifestyle and eating habits, it could be that you are undersecreting.

What to Do If You Feel You Are Low on Hydrochloric Acid

1 For a few days see if your symptoms improve if you eat small, frequent, low-protein high complex carbohydrate (whole grains, vegetables, fruit).
2 Chew all food thoroughly and don't eat when tired.
3 Don't drink water or anything with meals.
4 Wait for at least an hour before you have tea or coffee after a meal.
5 If symptoms persist, speak to a nutritionist (see Useful Addresses) and ask about a natural source of hydrochloric acid (betaine hydrochloride).
6 See if your doctor is willing to send you for a test to determine stomach acid levels. You will probably have to fast before a test. If your doctor cannot help you, ask to be referred to a doctor who specializes in Clinical Nutrition. The British Society of Nutritional Medicine (see Useful Addresses) will be able to give you the name of the doctor nearest to you. You could also ring a

nutritionist for advice. Biolab (see Useful Addresses) do the
Heidelberg Gastrogram Test. This entails swallowing a small
capsule at the end of a string which contains a microtransmitter.
The stomach acid levels are then recorded electronically.

Conditions Often Associated with Low Levels of Hydrochloric Acid

- *fatigue*
- *acne*
- *IBS*
- *food intolerances*
- *disturbances of gut flora*
- *pernicious anaemia*
- *asthma*
- *rheumatoid arthritis*
- *low immune system*

Food Intolerances

It has been said that one of the main causes of food intolerances is
faulty digestion in the stomach. This needs to be looked at first and
before embarking on drastic exclusion diets, which can cause
dramatic weight loss and severely affect the immune system and the
nervous system. Try simply cutting out junk foods and eating a
clean, well-balanced rotational diet. Cleansing the colon can also be
very helpful. (Send for 'The New Colon Cleansing Programme and
Beyond' from Higher Nature, price at the time of writing 30 pence.)

If the bowel is inflamed you might have to go very gently with
your cleansing programme. All the nutritionists in the Useful
Addresses section can give expert advice on colon cleansing and
can supply you with the necessary products. Describe your
symptoms carefully and remember that self-help programmes
should not be embarked upon before you have had a firm diagnosis
from your doctor.

Some people find Medical Herbalists or practitioners of Chinese
Medicine very helpful for cleansing the colon of old faeces.

7

IBS and Everyday Poisons

Before cleaning the colon is discussed, it is useful to look at some of the everyday poisons to which we subject our bodies.

Caffeine Allergy/Addiction

If you are fit and well you will probably be able to tolerate small daily amounts of tea and coffee without any trouble, but many people do not realize how they are affecting their bodies when they drink endless cups of tea and coffee day after day. Make an effort to cut down, particularly if you have allergies, digestive or nervous problems, cystitis or the restless legs syndrome (that awful feeling also known as 'singing legs' when your legs won't relax and you feel the need to move them even when you are in bed). You might have no trouble at all in giving up tea and coffee completely for a while, or even for good, but it is important to note that some people do experience great difficulties when they attempt this, and strangely enough it is not always people who are heavy tea, coffee or cola drinkers who suffer. In susceptible people, cutting down on caffeine can induce lethargy, and total abstinence can result in nausea, severe headaches, muscle and joint pains, and depression.

A Nasty Headache

The reason for this is the 'Caffeine Storm'; when the body is denied the drug, all the caffeine which has been stored in the body is released into the blood stream, and in effect causes a form of caffeine poisoning. The resulting headache is particularly severe, and in fact caffeine addicts are used to test the efficacy of headache drugs. Typically, as soon as tea or coffee is taken even in a small amount the headache eases, but the same cannot be said for the depression which often accompanies caffeine withdrawal. Some people feel down for several days. Occasionally after complete withdrawal, the depression can last for months. Homoeopathic treatment for caffeine addiction can be helpful, or mild symptoms can often be relieved by putting a grain of coffee or a couple of drops of tea under the tongue. The above information is not meant to discourage you from cleaning some of the caffeine out of your system – on the contrary, your bowel, kidneys and nervous system would welcome this – it has been included to help you to understand that some of the everyday things we drink are powerful drugs and some people will experience drug withdrawal symptoms; cut down slowly if you are one of the unlucky ones. You can do this by mixing decaffeinated coffee with your usual blend then increasing the amount of it until you are drinking all decaffeinated. If you drink filter instead of instant coffee you get fewer solids.

Stopping Smoking

There is no doubt that smoking injures the health and it would be a wonderful world if nobody smoked: cleaner and safer. All the NHS money that now goes on smoking-related diseases could go into other areas of medicine. Smoking is a pernicious addiction because it both calms and stimulates the nervous system. It is possibly because of this, and also the masked allergy factor, that some people find giving up so difficult. (A hidden or masked allergy can happen with *any* substance which is taken into the body daily; when the body is denied the substance the symptoms appear. This is explained fully in *A Little Bit of What You Fancy* by Dr Richard Mackarness, published by Pan.)

Why Some People Fail Repeatedly

Some people give up smoking without any problems at all; they just stop. Others crave cigarettes and feel they don't know what to do with their hands, but can distract themselves with a cup of coffee, eating sweets or doing something active. These two groups often scorn the person who fails again and again to give up the awful weed, and proclaim loudly that it is just a matter of will-power. Will-power certainly comes into it, and for those who do not suffer physical or psychological symptoms perhaps it is all that is needed to stop; but for the physically addicted/allergic smoker, there is a lot more to it – lack of will-power or weakness cannot be the cause of swollen joints, skin problems, and so on.

Severe Nicotine Withdrawal

For some people there is a clearly defined withdrawal syndrome (a collection of symptoms) when they abstain from nicotine. This is not surprising because the drug affects many systems in the body and it is just like giving up heroin, tranquillizers or any other addictive substance. Common complaints are:

- *Feeling anxious and depressed*
- *Irritability*
- *Headaches*
- *Being unable to think clearly*
- *Being unable to think of simple words*
- *Constipation*
- *Sugar craving*
- *Coffee craving*
- *Aching joints and muscles*
- *Extreme fatigue*
- *Swelling of the face*
- *Rashes*
- *Persistent coughs*
- *Chest infections*

- *Asthma attacks*
- *Sore throats*

People who have tried several times to stop smoking know these feelings very well, they even know which symptoms will come in the first week and how long it takes for the joint pains to start and so on; unfortunately, they also know how quickly the symptoms go when they resume smoking.

Reasons for Failure

Lack of information heads this list; if people know what to expect and are reassured that the feelings will not last forever, they stand a much better chance of succeeding. Also if they prepare their bodies for the trauma – and make no mistake, it can take its toll physically – the chances of success are further improved.

Some 'Stop Smoking' Books Are Not Worth Reading

Many people are discouraged when they read books which don't even begin to describe what they are going through, and because some of the more severe effects are not mentioned they begin to think there is something else wrong with them. Don't read books that pat you on the head and tell you to go for a walk, take a glass of water, or reach for your macramé every time you crave a fag; realize it is going to be difficult and accept it. You will be rewarded. You may never forget the pleasure of a cigarette, but the relief of being a non-smoker will dull that memory. You will feel healthier (eventually), cleaner, smell nicer, and enjoy your food much more – eating will no longer be just the thing you do before having coffee and a cigarette. Life also becomes much more leisurely, nicotine craving does not dictate where you sit when you travel or when you take a break from work; when you stop smoking *you* are in charge.

Preparing to Stop

If you are an addictive smoker you are likely to have unstable blood sugar levels. Read chapter 17 carefully and adjust your diet accordingly. *If your blood sugar is allowed to drop you are ten times more likely to beg someone for a cigarette.* Keep a bag of sunflower seeds in your pocket and at first eat some every hour between meals. They are full of good things and will keep your blood sugar levels stable. Another way in which diet can help you is to eat foods which leave an alkaline residue or ash when they are broken down in the body; vegetables, particularly raw and the less sweet fruits are good. Research has shown an overacid body is more likely to crave cigarettes.

You Need More Than a Good Diet

Take an honest look at your nutritional state and build your body up for the coming stress. Every cigarette you smoke robs you of 25 mg of vitamin C, so you are bound to be short of this; your requirements for vitamin C and all nutrients rise sharply when your body is under siege. Taking large quantities of certain nutrients is not very helpful since they often depend upon each other for absorption. One way around this is to take both a good quality combined multivitamin and multimineral preparation. If you feel you can identify any particular deficiency you can take an additional supply of that mineral or vitamin. A good book that could help you pinpoint your deficiencies is *Nutritional Medicine* by Dr Stephen Davies and Dr Alan Stewart (published by Pan).

Which Supplements Will Help?

Vitamin C has long been known to aid detoxification, strengthen the immune system and ease withdrawal symptoms. Vitamin B_3 – niacin – has also been found to be helpful. This chemical, which can also be bought in the form of nicotinic acid, is similar in structure to nicotine. Niacin is also thought to resemble endogenous benzodiazepine – a tranquillizing substance similar to Valium made naturally in the brain. In the United States large quantities of niacin are used in detoxification programmes. Its use is combined with saunas and exercise and seems to have wonderful results, and there appear to be few toxic effects even at very high dosages. The usual recommended dose is to build up to 100 mg morning and 100 mg at night. Don't be surprised if your skin pricks and you go bright red twenty minutes or so after taking it; this is a harmless flush and is beneficial. Niacin improves circulation to the extremities (it is used for chilblains and Raynaud's Disease, a condition characterized by cold, white or blue fingers, caused by spasm in the arteries in the hands), and acts like an internal sauna. It is also known to be essential to the health of the bowel. People who are always cold often find this supplement helpful and many people say that after the first few doses they feel very much calmer. The only thing to remember is to take all the B vitamins if you take this; no B vitamin should be taken in isolation because it depletes the store of the others.

Experienced nutritional advice for Irritable Bowel Syndrome and other colon problems is available from New Nutrition – see Useful Addresses, page 210.

Encouraging Experiences

Alan had been a moderate smoker for twenty years. He has now been a non-smoker for four years and says he never gives cigarettes a thought. He felt his previous attempts had failed through lack of information and attempting to give up when he was under stress. Each time he tried it was lack of concentration and feeling far away that made him start again; he felt his work was suffering. When he had to go into hospital for a hernia repair he decided this was a good time to stop; he would be able to slow down for several weeks.

He had never had chest problems but coughed a lot the first few weeks. It cleared his chest but was rather painful because of his abdominal stitches. He recovered well from the surgery but felt far away and not very interested in things for three months. After that he felt fine.

Margery had been a heavy smoker for ten years. She gave up two years ago. She had tried for a year to give up and the longest she lasted was three weeks (the famous three week crisis). She had no trouble with craving (some people don't), but feeling depressed and 'ill all over' drove her back each time.

Before one Christmas she was made redundant and decided she could not feel much worse; it was a good time to try again. She ate lots of Christmas fare, chocolates, nuts and fruit and had more than her one sherry before dinner. Her glands and joints swelled and ached and she felt very depressed. She also had a few panic attacks; this had not happened before. After she got past the third week she knew she would make it but it was six months before she really felt herself. She has never regretted stopping and still feels it was like coming out of prison.

Nick had not realized it was going to be difficult to stop smoking, in fact, he was one of the 'Oh, it's easy, I can stop any time I like' smokers. The reality of the situation was quite different; after two unsuccesful attempts he asked his doctor for Nicorette gum. He found this a great help although when he used it the way the packaging suggested – keeping a piece in his cheek and slowly chewing on it from time to time – it gave him a sore mouth. This problem was solved by cutting the gum into quarters and chewing it normally with a piece of ordinary mint gum; it tasted better too. A cup of coffee (see below) and the gum after meals was his lifeline for two months, and then he gradually forgot about the Nicorette. He had a few panic attacks (this is not uncommon even after being symptom-free for about six months) but he revealed his 'silly episodes' to a friend and found he had had the same experience when he gave up smoking. He was very constipated and, in fact, dates his Irritable Bowel problems from that time.

Going 'Cold Turkey' or Cutting Down Slowly?

It is worth noting that if you cut down by any more than a third of the daily amount of cigarettes you could have a full-blown withdrawal syndrome even though you are still smoking. Maybe this is why total abstinence is usually encouraged. On the other hand if you could gradually cut down without lapsing when you had a night out or a bad day, and look after your diet and so on, it could make the final bid easier. It is to be hoped that you will take heart from these stories and remember at the time these people gave up they knew nothing about diet or supplements – you are going to find it much easier!

Smoking and Caffeine

The *British Medical Journal* published some material which shows that caffeine metabolism slows down within days of giving up smoking. Smokers often tend to be quite heavy coffee drinkers, possibly because they metabolize caffeine faster. If they continue with the same amount after the caffeine metabolism slows down, their blood levels of caffeine may go up by 250 per cent. This can continue for several months after stopping smoking. It would seem sensible to change to decaffeinated coffee and even to cut down on that before stopping smoking. Caffeine poisoning could be a large part of the unpleasantness of withdrawal for some people.

The Cup that Cheers

By now you will probably feel like using this book for firelighters – one deprivation after another, you might say. 'Does alcohol have to go too? I don't drink much.' Only temporarily; when your bowel has recovered you could resume moderate drinking habits if you wish, except of course if you are known to be allergic to it, or if you have had a drinking problem in the past.

Alcohol and the Irritable Bowel Syndrome

It is unrealistic to expect bowel symptoms to improve until you have given up alcohol. Apart from feeding *Candida* and making blood sugar levels unstable, it also interferes with the absorption of nutrients essential for the healthy functioning of the bowel.

Alcoholism

Reactions to alcohol vary in a similar way to reactions to nicotine or tranquillizers, in that some people can just stop – even after years of heavy drinking – and have no problems, while others are dramatically physically and emotionally ill when they abstain.

The Withdrawal Syndrome

While it is acknowledged that there is a definite alcohol withdrawal syndrome, much of what is written about it does not give a true picture. For example, the physical effects of alcohol withdrawal are usually said to be over in three weeks. Some of them have not even *started* then – the muscle spasm may not appear until the sixth or eighth week.

Alcoholism is often treated as a psychological, sociological or moral problem. No doubt problems in these areas can co-exist but since the nutritional treatment approach is so successful, the primary cause must be physical. The failure of the conventional treatment methods for alcoholism must be because so many professionals refuse to see the condition as the disease it so patently is. Everybody agrees it is characterized by loss of control and excessive drinking, but this is often the last thing in the world the sufferer actually wants. What is happening in his body that keeps him in this state?

Body Chemistry and Alcoholism

In the past forty years, research has linked alcoholism to biochemistry in various ways.

The Masked Allergy Theory

Allergy and addiction were thought to be different reactions but recent research suggests that the only difference is in the timing of the symptoms.

Low Blood Sugar and Alcoholism

It is well known that recovering alcoholics crave sugary foods. Increasing evidence is showing that many alcoholics have shown symptoms of faulty sugar metabolism since childhood.

Caffeine and Alcohol

Caffeine is another substance which gives temporary relief to the symptoms of low blood sugar and it is possibly because of this that heavy drinkers often drink cola, tea and coffee during the day and alcohol in the evenings. The caffeine eases the low blood sugar symptoms (a large part of the misery of a hangover) until the evening drinking starts and so the circle continues. This would fit with the theory that alcoholics have nutritional deficiencies before becoming alcoholics and that while in part their nutritional deficiencies are due to mal-absorption caused by alcohol, some degree of deficiency precedes the drinking.

Alcohol and Heredity

It could be argued that bad character traits can be inherited – so can biochemical make-up.

Nutritional Requirements and Alcoholism

The desire for alcohol may begin with stress and each drink taken depletes the body's store of nutrients. Though alcohol has plenty of calories it has no food value (the large abdomen and thin arms and legs of many drinkers confirms this) and also the burning up of the alcohol in itself further reduces the food in the body's storehouse. So by the time the effect on the bowel is considered it is a wonder that any nutrients at all are absorbed.

How Does a Good Diet Help?

Animal studies have shown that voluntary alcohol consumption can be repeatedly turned on and off by giving the animals different diets. Those with a balanced, vitamin rich diet choose less, while those with a poor diet which has been reduced in carbohydrate and fat, choose more.

Treatment by Diet

This includes keeping to a very strict low blood sugar diet and including vitamin and mineral supplements. Again vitamins C and B₃ have been found to be very helpful and doses much larger than for other conditions are used. In addition the simple food supplement L-glutamine, an amino acid, has been found greatly to reduce the discomfort of alcohol withdrawal.* Whole grains and pulses are also useful both as a source of protein and to stabilize the blood sugar levels. If liver damage has already occurred animal protein may not be tolerated.

Alcohol as an Emotional Painkiller

Not every problem drinker starts with a biochemical defect. Because it is an emotional anaesthetic some people use it to blot out the pain of the past or present. Unfortunately this only adds more problems; the self-esteem of sufferers drops even further, they despise themselves for lack of control, suffer from guilt and on top of all this they have the harmful physical effects to cope with. There is no easy way to cope with painful memories, difficulties in the present and fear of the future. You can only start by accepting and loving yourself exactly as you are and acknowledging that pain hurts; you would not be trying to numb the feelings if they weren't too painful to bear. We start doing this as little children, we overbreathe, tighten our muscles with tension or switch off into depression if life hurts too much. (There is more on this subject in my book *Coping with Anxiety and Depression*, published by Sheldon Press).

* Offprint on L-Glutamine, The Surprising Brain Fuel, available from Higher Nature, price 30 pence. See Useful Addresses.

Counselling and Support

The recovery rate is higher in people who attend Alcoholics Anonymous and similar organizations than it is for those who have had medical treatment. The human warmth and spiritual teaching of AA has been a lifeline to countless people. You will find the number of your local group in the telephone book.

For the nutritional approach to addictions, nervousness and panic attacks read *No More Fears*, by Dr Douglas Hunt (published by Thorsons).

8

The Bowel as a Dumping Ground

Some people treat their digestive tract like a rubbish disposal system and give little thought to the damage caused by the careless diet. When the colon is irritated by diet, stress, drugs, chemicals, and so on, it tries to protect itself by producing more mucus. This can bind with the sludge from refined foods, such as white flour, and build up on the wall of the bowel the way silt builds up in a river. This layer of gluey hardened faeces can weigh several pounds, and is a good place for harmful organisms to breed. It also prevents the complete absorption of nutrients by preventing digested food coming into contact with the lining of the bowel. The production of *digestive enzymes*, chemicals necessary to break down the food for complete absorption, is also affected.

How Does a Dirty Colon Affect the Body?

The local effects of this poisonous residue are irritation and inflammation. The general effects include:

- *diarrhoea*
- *constipation*
- *fatigue*

- *headaches*
- *dull eyes*
- *poor skin*
- *spots*
- *aching muscles*
- *joint pains*
- *depression*

This is because the poisons go through a network of vessels called the lymphatic system to all parts of the body; the equivalent of dirty dish-water is carried around the body, instead of a clean, nourishing fluid, the function of which should be to feed cells not served by blood vessels. The lymphatic fluid also kills off harmful organisms and carries away the refuse.

If the body has to battle against these poisons long-term, it is not surprising that it sometimes has to give up and the disease process takes over – the result is inflammation, infection and degeneration. It is understandable that there are more and more people referred to hospitals for Irritable Bowel Syndrome, colitis (inflammation of the colon), Crohn's disease (inflammation of the small intestine), colon cancer and diverticulosis.

Diverticulitis

When the muscles of the colon wall have to work overtime to deal with hard stools or lack of bulk in the diet, they become weakened and lose their elasticity. This causes pouches called *Diverticula*. The food trapped in these pockets makes wonderful breeding ground for bacteria. The result can be *Diverticulitis*, an infection where there is often a fever and acute abdominal pain. This condition needs medical help.

Diverticula Disease/Irritable Bowel Syndrome

Where symptoms are not severe and are treated by the GP these two diagnoses are often interchangeable. Men are more likely to be told they have diverticula problems, women are more likely to be told they have Irritable Bowel Syndrome.

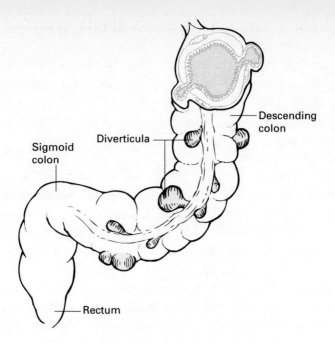

Fig. 2. Section of colon showing diverticula

Spring Cleaning the Bowel

When they become aware of the dangers of a dirty colon, some people become too enthusiastic and embark on drastic colon cleansing programmes which can result in poisons pouring into the bloodstream and although the final result is very beneficial the process can make the sufferer feel wretched. The experience of detoxification can entail:

- *migraine*
- *blinding headaches*
- *nausea*
- *flu-like symptoms*
- *aches and pains*
- *fever*
- *exhaustion*
- *anxiety*

- *panic attacks*
- *irritability*
- *weepiness*
- *sometimes quite profound depression.*

This can be avoided by taking it slowly, flushing the poisons out a little at a time.

Where Do I Start?

Simply by cleaning up your diet. Cut down on foods which are collecting on the walls of the bowel: refined flours, sugar, cakes, biscuits, refined cereals, fatty foods. Increase the foods which are going to act as gentle scouring pads as they go through the gut: vegetables raw and cooked; fruit, fresh stewed or dried; whole grains and pulses; seeds and nuts. Every time you reach out for a snack, possibly one which has comforted you since childhood, perhaps a piece of white bread or a doughnut, imagine trying to use it to clean out a sticky bowl, then imagine cleaning out the same bowl with a handful of fibrous raw vegetables or chewy brown rice.

Food and Security

People often become anxious or even aggressive when a change of eating habits is suggested; here are some typical comments:
But sugar gives me energy; I need it. It always makes me feel better.
Sugar has no nutritional value; it is empty calories. Yes, it can give you energy temporarily but it does more harm than good in the long term. See page 113 on blood sugar levels.

But I must have some bread. I could never feel full without it; everybody needs it – it is the staff of life.

Wholemeal bread is very good food but for some people wheat and yeast can be the source of major problems (page 88).

But I've always missed breakfast, had a sandwich at lunchtime and a big meal in the evening.

This is an unhealthy way to eat, expecting your body to function without fuel during your working hours. It can cause fatigue, tension, irritability and overweight.

But that's not a proper meal…

What is a Proper Meal?

Some people cling to the idea that a nutritious meal must be of a mixture of protein and starch, such as: steak pie, cabbage, potatoes and gravy, or fish, peas and chips. Not only is it unnecessary to eat this way but it can also put a great strain on the digestive system. Research has shown that starch – bread, potatoes, sugar – and protein – meat, fish, eggs and poultry – require different gastric juices for digestion, so if they are eaten together, neither food has the medium necessary to break it down efficiently, digestion is slowed down, and gas, bloating and indigestion can result. This is explained fully in *Food Combining for Health: Don't Mix Foods That Fight* by Doris Grant and Jean Joice, (published by Thorsons).
It can be very liberating for you and your digestive system to give up old-fashioned ideas. If your diet is varied it is perfectly sound nutrition to eat nothing but apples or grains or vegetables for a meal as long as you eat enough. Proper meals are adequate amounts of a variety of clean foods.

Cleaning Up the Diet

Note: any dietary suggestions contained in this book are only for people who are overweight or the correct weight for their height and build. People who have a diet from their doctor or people who have ever had an eating disorder or severe depression must consult their doctor before changing their eating habits.

How Long Does it Take to Clean the Colon?

The debris has been collecting for years, so it is unlikely you will have a pristine inside in a couple of weeks. It could take months.

You will know when things are happening; your skin and eyes will look clearer, your digestion will improve, you will have more energy and niggling aches and pains which have been around for years will disappear. You could feel mentally better too, less jumpy, and clearer-headed.

Some people say it feels like grief having to give up their favourite foods, but at the same time they are so delighted by the change in their appearance they are willing to resist a tasty hamburger or a bowl of English toffee icecream.

Stage One

Note: this is a clean-up diet rather than an elimination diet for allergies, but in fact some people have found that after cleansing the bowel, if they combine foods carefully they can tolerate foods which had previously caused trouble. Also note you are not going to feel good initially, in fact as you detoxify you could feel tired and heavy-limbed. Some people experience a furred tongue, nausea and joint pains. This is why cleaning out in stages has been suggested. Try to stay with it; the feelings pass in a few days and remember the worse you feel the cleaner you are becoming inside.

Getting Started

Think about what you are putting in your mouth; has it been messed about? Does it contain chemicals? What has been lost in the processing? How is it packaged? Do you really want to eat dyes, or munch snacks covered with large quantities of salt to conceal the fact that they have been cooked in rancid fat? *Your body is just not built to cope with this.*

GIVE UP:

1   *Regular consumption of junk foods*
2   *All dairy products (except live yogurt), even for a month; these are the main cause of allergic problems in infants and adults so it makes sense to start here.*

This request usually brings cries of protest, 'But how can I live without cheese or milk' – you can, and you will be surprised how quickly the desire for these foods will go. You could substitute goat's or sheep's milk, yogurt and cheese. Some people use soya milk for drinking, cooking and making yogurt.

CUT DOWN:

3   *Tea, coffee, chocolate and all soft drinks (see page 38).*
4   *Alcohol. Make sure you eat fruit or drink fruit juice at the time you would normally have an alcoholic drink.*

Increase 'Dredger Food'

1   *Wholegrains: oats, brown rice, barley, millet, rye*
2   *Pulses: lentils, beans, peas*
3   *Fruit and vegetables including sea vegetables (sounds better than seaweed)*
4   *Fish, olive oil, sunflower oil*
5   *Nuts (not peanuts) and seeds*
6   *Take water, fruit juice, herb teas or coffee substitute at some of your tea breaks.*

Stage Two

You might be ready for this after a week but if you are still struggling continue stage one for another week.

CUT DOWN:

1   *Meat, eggs, and poultry*
2   *Tea, coffee, soft drinks and alcohol more than in stage one.*

Increase Whole Clean Foods

More vegetables, fruit, grains as in stage one.

Stage Three

On paper this is going to look depressing, but when you are up to stage three you should be used to being deprived. (Although hearty bowls of lentil and vegetable soup, or baked potatoes with nut butter or yogurt and herbs, curried vegetables and rice or pasta tossed in olive oil with garlic mushrooms and tomatoes is not exactly starvation rations, is it?)

EAT ONLY:

Whole grains, vegetables, sea vegetables, fruit: fresh or dried, nuts, seeds, olive oil or sunflower oil, or products made from any of these if they do not contain additives.

DRINK:

Water, bottled or filtered if possible, fruit juices preferably diluted, bancha tea, herb teas, coffee substitutes or, if you cannot make it without, one cup of weak tea or filtered coffee per day.

Your Hard Work Will Be Rewarded

By now you might be ready to rush out for fish and chips to settle your nerves – don't despair and think what you will gain:

1 *The bowel will work more efficiently, the absorption sites will be cleared, enzyme production will increase and as a result your bowel should be less irritable.*
2 *Because you have eaten less concentrated protein you will have been eating better combinations of foods. Also your kidneys and liver will have been rested.*
3 *Because of reducing your sugar intake your pancreas will be less strained and your blood sugar levels should be more stable.*
4 *You will probably have lost some excess weight or puffiness.*
5 *You will look healthier.*

Getting Back to a Normal Diet

Introduce foods one at a time, and notice if you feel uncomfortable or down with any of them, or if any symptoms such as aching joints, a stuffy nose or headaches reappear. If this happens restrict the offending food to once every four days. If symptoms persist, please consult a doctor trained in food allergy treatment.

Stimulating the Skin to Get Rid of Poisons

While the digestive tract and the kidneys are the main organs of excretion, the skin has also a very important part to play; it is a great deal more useful than just a waterproof covering that keeps our bits and pieces together. If it is kept healthy it can be a wonderful waste disposal system. It covers such a large area it is worth getting it to work for you.

Sweating it Out

A fever is nature's way of helping us to lose toxins through the skin. You can stimulate sweating with some water therapies.

Water Therapy

Regular swimming is very beneficial; steam baths, saunas and jacuzzis also encourage detoxification.

Caution: consult your doctor before using water treatments if you have heart trouble, high blood pressure, diabetes, epilepsy or any condition which might be aggravated by extremes of temperature.

Salt Baths

These encourage detoxification and greatly help muscle and joint pains. Add 2 lbs of salt or three cupfuls of Epsom salts to a comfortably hot bath and lie in it for twenty minutes; add hot water as it cools. If you drink a pint of hot honey and lemon, or peppermint tea while you soak it will further encourage sweating. A cold flannel on the forehead might make you feel more comfortable. The next step is to wrap up in cotton towels and get into a warm bed. You should perspire freely and sleep well. If you have to bathe during the day finish with a cold shower and rest for half an hour. You could do this three times weekly.

Foot Baths

For aching feet and to stimulate circulation use alternating bowls of hot and cold water, staying two minutes in each; carry on for about twenty minutes. If you like you could add one cup of salt or ½ cup of Epsom salts to the hot water. When you have finished wrap the feet in a towel and lie down for half an hour.

Skin Brushing

This stimulates the lymphatic system (see page 51), and involves brushing all over with a natural bristle brush for about ten minutes before you shower or bath. Start with the soles of the feet and work on all areas except broken skin, the face, neck and breasts. It can be boring but the results are worth it. In addition to elimination toxins, because circulation is increased, it will also improve the texture of your skin. Boots, Higher Nature and the Body Shop have skin brushes or you might have an old hairbrush that would do the job; wash it carefully.

The Experience of Others

Suzi had suffered with a swollen face, mental dullness, headaches and visual disturbances periodically since she was a child. When she was 24 she saw a nutrition counsellor who explained about the Toxic Colon Syndrome. She gave up tea, coffee and alcohol and lived on vegetables, fruit, beans, lentils, whole grains, nuts, seeds, goat's milk and soya products for a month. She felt sick and had headaches for the first two days then she felt progressively better; she lost weight, her face did not swell, she was mentally clearer and her eyesight improved. She has kept to the basic diet but has included fish, chicken and eggs. While cleaning up her diet has changed her life she has not become obsessive about it and lapses at holiday times. Her symptoms return if she does this for too long.

Pete's digestion had been upset for three years, ever since he suffered an attack of diarrhoea while on holiday abroad. He complained of bloating, constipation, discomfort after certain foods and insomnia. After full gastroenterological tests he was diagnosed as having the Irritable Bowel Syndrome. He was given a high-fibre diet and anti-spasmodic drugs, but did not improve. He was not convinced when the value of the raw food diet was explained to him; he argued that since he could not digest cooked vegetables he was unlikely to digest them raw. He gave up dairy produce, cut down on coffee and alcohol and started a 70 per cent raw food diet. He took time over his meals and chewed them well. His digestion did not improve in the first week and he was beginning to get discouraged when he noticed a rash he had had on his legs for months had completely cleared up. He continued with the diet and within a month was feeling much better. He keeps well if he combines foods carefully and includes lots of salads and fruit. How the enzymes in raw food aid digestion is fully explained in *Raw Energy*, by Leslie and Susannah Kenton (Century Arrow).

9

IBS and the Nervous System

The cause of the Irritable Bowel Syndrome might be overgrowth of candida in one person, a toxic colon in another. Another cause is one that many sufferers stubbornly refuse to acknowledge – an exhausted nervous system. They search and search for something 'physical' when the cause of the trouble is right under their noses, but what could be more physical than overstimulated nerves? They are part of the body too. In order to understand how tired nerves affect the bowel it is necessary to have some idea of how the nervous system works.

Understanding the Nervous System

The nervous system can be compared to a railway network; it provides lines of communication between various parts of the body, with the brain as the central station, the spine as the main line and the supply to the hands and feet as the branch lines. It is divided into the central nervous system and the autonomic nervous system.

The Central Nervous System

This controls voluntary movement and is responsible for all sensations in muscles, bones and joints. It is under the control of the *will* – you want to pick up a cup, you reach out your hand and do so. This system works well unless it is neurologically impaired or, in times of terror, paralysed with fear.

The Autonomic Nervous System

The autonomic nervous system controls all involuntary muscles, including internal organs, and blood vessels. This system is under the control of the emotions, for example, anger will cause your blood pressure to rise, fear will make the stomach churn. It has two parts: the sympathetic nervous system, which has a stimulating effect, and the parasympathetic, which has a calming effect. *When your parasympathetic nervous system does not work properly you become overanxious.*

Think of the sympathetic nervous system as the express trains speeding along and the parasympathetic nervous system as the slow trains pottering along, taking time and enjoying the view. All the internal organs have two sets of nerves, one stimulating, the other quietening – remember this important point when you are arguing with your bowel.

The Sympathetic Nervous System

Imagine you are walking across a field; a bull crashes through the fence and charges. You are terrified and your nervous system is 'sympathetic' to these emotions and prepares your body to fight for survival. It does this in response to you *tightening* your muscles and squeezing your glands – and rather like squeezing oranges it produces 'juice'. This juice is a chemical called adrenalin. As a result, your blood pressure rises, your heart rate speeds up, breathing becomes rapid (you need more oxygen because you are rushing around) and you sweat to cool off. To help even more, your blood is diverted from the abdomen to the legs so that you can run faster.

This is the reason for that sinking feeling in the tummy when we are afraid. With a reduced blood supply to your digestive organs you do not think of food, or of the need to go to the lavatory. So when your sympathetic nervous system is in action, your *adrenalin/anxiety levels are high*.

In this situation, the body is behaving very much like that of an over-anxious person – rapid breathing and pulse, sweating and so on. The difference is that the anxiety is being used productively, because there *is* something to worry about. Sometimes the body becomes so scared that vomiting is induced, together with the emptying of the bowel and bladder (shit-scared – another point to remember). This may be a primitive mechanism for making the body lighter to enable it to run faster.

What Happens When the Danger is Over?

When you escape from the bull and are sitting in the farmhouse having a cup of tea, all you need to do to switch off the extra adrenalin that is still making your pulse race is to *relax* your tight muscles. This releases chemicals which turn off the supply of adrenalin. This is the *parasympathetic nervous system* working efficiently; the blood pressure drops, the heart rate and breathing slow down, you stop sweating, the blood comes back into your abdomen from your arms and legs – you realize you are hungry. You are also conscious that you need the lavatory. You feel relaxed; your muscles are comfortable. So then your *adrenalin/anxiety levels are low*.

It is easy to see from this example why the nerves get exhausted. Repeated stresses, conscious and unconscious (even small ones), keep us in a state of red alert all the time. It's like someone continually running away from a non-existent bull; they want to slow down but they can't. Their adrenalin (and therefore anxiety) levels are still too high. Have you ever been so wound up that you carried on working long after you need to even though you were exhausted?

Nervous Diarrhoea

Nervous diarrhoea is frequent loose bowel movements not caused by infection, irritation or food allergy. It can be one urgent movement on waking, or several small movements throughout the day. These can be with or without pain and they can often leave the sufferer exhausted.

Nervous diarrhoea is caused by the nerves to the bowel getting the wrong messages. When the red alert button is pressed and the sympathetic nervous system springs into action, at first the message is to suspend activity in the bowel, but if the message carries on too long and becomes 'I'm very scared', instead of, 'I need to act', so much adrenalin is poured in that the bowel opens. This is what is happening in nervous diarrhoea – the body is so hyped-up that the bowel cannot relax. Some people have to rush up each morning with diarrhoea – their parasympathetic nervous system is still too active even when they sleep.

Is your bowel responding as though you were running from the charging bull all the time? If so, you are the only one who can do anything about this. The behaviour of your boss, your spouse or worry over money may be your 'charging bull' but whatever it is no person or situation can affect your nervous system unless you allow them to do so. As far as relationships go, if you have openly and honestly *declared* to the person concerned that you find their behaviour to you distressing, then it is up to you after that. If you spend your time trying to make those around you change then you are in for a frustrating time and you deserve diarrhoea. On the other hand if you change your reaction to the stress and look after your body in spite of it, you will realize that far from the action of your bowel being out of your control, you can learn how to restore it to normal functioning.

Fear of Not Making the Lavatory in Time

Your diarrhoea may be so bad that you are afraid to go out of the house, or only if you plan a route where you have access to a lavatory several times on the way. You are on the treadmill of fear– diarrhoea, fear–diarrhoea. If you are constantly sending fearful messages to the bowel, the diarrhoea will continue. You could take a diarrhoea mixture to give you more confidence for special occasions but the essential treatment is to change the message to the bowel – this is the only permanent treatment. You are the only one who can heal your nervous system and don't be surprised if there are ups and downs, nature does not heal in a straight line. Help with this is on page 120 but you could also try delaying the call to stool. When you have the urge to go to the lavatory practise hanging on: even if you can only manage two seconds, keep trying and you will gradually gain more control. Stand or sit on a chair outside the lavatory, breathe slowly, tighten your buttocks and start to count on your fingers squeezing each one hard. You could do something similar when you are out too; count how many steps you can go past the lavatory before you double back.

Since there is a good clean out in the mornings or several stools per day the amount of faeces on these panic visits is small. Although people with this problem are rarely incontinent outdoors it might make you feel safer if you protected yourself against the possibility. You could line your underpants or knickers with plastic and then cover that with tissue, kitchen roll, cotton wool or sanitary towels. Boots sell baby pants that are just a piece of plastic without elastic, or you could cut a plastic carrier bag to the shape you want. You may throw up your hands in horror and say you would rather stay indoors, but think about it; *who but you would know?* After all it is a temporary state, but when your nerves are better your diarrhoea will be a thing of the past. Get your mind out of your bowel and stop giving it all those negative commands: 'I'll never make the loo,' 'I can't go out because of the diarrhoea,' and so on.

Vicky had been housebound with fear of incontinence outside for two years, then one day the person who normally collected her children from school rang to say she was delayed and could not make it in time. Vicky was panic-stricken but knew she would have to go. The school was only two streets away and she delayed leaving the house until the last minute. As she rushed out of the gate she turned her ankle on the step, the pain was severe and she had to hobble to the school. It was not until she was back home that she realized that she had not given her diarrhoea a thought; her bowel had had a rest from worrying messages because her thoughts were concentrated on the pain of her ankle.

While the nerves of the internal organs are not normally under the control of the will you can train yourself to have some degree of control, and change the functioning of any organ of your body. See chapter 18 on biofeedback and autogenic training.

Nervous Constipation

This has the same cause as nervous diarrhoea except that the train receives a different signal, so to speak. This time the instructions say 'Tight muscles ahead, slow down activity'. You will remember that the initial instructions of the person preparing to run were, 'I need more blood in my arms and legs so take the blood from my digestive system; I do not need it there at the moment.' Tense people get stuck in this situation, tight muscles all over including the abdomen.

The Relaxation Response

Healthy people are able to use their minds and bodies to full capacity and then when they are ready to relax they just switch off – their relaxation response is in working order. The relaxation response in people who are tense and nervously exhausted fails because it has been overworked. Before it will function normally again it needs some help. Here is a less dramatic scene than the charging bull to help you to understand why the nervous system eventually stops trying to cope with the extra load.

The Adrenalin Event

Two men are going for a run. One is in track one, the other is in track two. Imagine they are both wearing red vests. Extra energy is needed to run, so in response to their thought, 'I am going to run,' the brain sends a message for the muscles to contract and this squeezes the glands which produce adrenalin. Thoughts, heart-rate and breathing rate increase, blood is diverted from the internal organs to the legs to allow them to move faster; everything speeds up. The adrenalin levels are high. The two men complete the circuit and prepare to go home.

The Man in Track One. This man's muscles relax and in response to this, chemicals which oppose adrenalin are released into the bloodstream. His heart-rate and breathing slow down, everything goes back to normal. His adrenalin levels are falling – imagine he has showered and is now wearing a blue vest. When he arrives home he is hungry and needs the bathroom. After dinner he repairs his son's bicycle, watches television and then goes to bed and sleeps like a baby. When he awakes he feels rested.

The Man in Track Two. Because he has been overworking lately his relaxation response is worn out. After the run his muscles do not automatically relax, so he is deprived of the chemicals which would slow him down; his adrenalin levels have not gone down. When he arrives home, although he has showered and gone through the same motions as the other man, it is as if he is still wearing the *red* vest. He is preoccupied with worrying thoughts, he is irritable with his kids, his digestion feels upset (the extra blood is still in his legs), he does not want dinner, he tries to read the newspaper but can't concentrate. His evening is spent looking for antacid tablets, making frequent visits to the lavatory to pass urine, and chasing next door's cat from the flower borders. He has difficulty getting off to sleep; when he does he sleeps fitfully. At 3 a.m. he wakes feeling anxious and hungry; he sleeps again and in the morning he wakes feeling anxious and stiff and sore. His muscles are still not relaxed – his adrenalin levels are still high. And it could go on like this until he has a nervous breakdown, a heart attack or some illness which will force him to slow down, *unless* he gets wise and realizes that all he has to do to don a blue vest is to slow down – to practise *mechanically* what his body has given up doing *automatically*. He must re-educate his muscles through relaxation exercises and consciously gearing down.

The Irritable Bowel Syndrome and Insomnia

Many sufferers of IBS complain of insomnia although rarely is it due to actual pain. Many say they are aware of wind but it does not really cause discomfort, only a feeling of extreme wakefulness. Judith's story is typical:

I know by early evening what the night will bring. After my meal I start to feel restless and sometimes slightly uncomfortable in my tummy. When bed time comes my mind is weary and I long for sleep but I feel so wide awake. The pattern is so familiar now I just have to accept it. I get up and down and have a hot drink or a snack and then so predictably about 3 a.m. I can feel rumblings in my gut and – it is like someone pressing a switch – I can then fall asleep. I sometimes find that eating something quite substantial helps to speed the process up a bit. I also find that massaging my feet very firmly and – I know it sounds odd – having a cold shower and then getting back into a warm bed sometimes does the trick.

Judith's cold shower may not be such a strange idea; it is accepted that food allergy symptoms are much worse if you are hot. It is also understandable that the bowel can cause sleeplessness even when their is no discomfort; bacteria in the gut produce chemicals which make us sleepy, so if there is an imbalance in the gut flora this effect may be reduced.

Other causes of insomnia include excitement, worry, itching, pain, lack of exercise and fresh air and breathing problems.

What Can I Do?

It is unlikely that you will find anything that is consistently helpful other than taking good care of your nervous system. This begins when you get up in the morning. It is a mistake to habitually sleep late if you have a bad night. This disturbs the normal body rhythm and because you miss the effect of the light in the brightest part of the day you end up feeling jet-lagged all the time. You can always rest later in the day but force yourself out of bed and keep to a routine. Help with retraining your wayward nerves is in the self-help section of the book (page 120).

Stress Hormones and IBS

If the pancreas is under stress and secretes too much insulin this affects the output of several hormones, epinephrine, norepinephrine and adrenocorticotropin, which triggers the release of cortisol. This is produced in the adrenal glands and slows down the fat-burning process. During times of stress a significant portion of spare fat in the bloodstream goes to your abdomen for emergency use. This could be the reason why many anxious people feel they are gaining weight and changing shape even when their eating habits remain the same. High cortisol levels not only make you feel more anxious and deplete your immune system, leaving you more susceptible to infections, but also lower the production of another important hormone produced in the adrenal glands: DHEA – dehydroepiandrosterone (as discussed by Alan R Gaby, MD, *American Holistic Medicine*, Spring 1993, pages 19–23).

Until recent years, DHEA, a steroid hormone, has been given little attention. Formerly it was thought to be only a 'bank' on which the adrenal glands could draw to produce other hormones such as oestrogen and progesterone. Scientists have now shown that it has very important functions of its own. It may strengthen the immune system, and be of value in preventing heart disease, diabetes, cancer,

Alzheimer's disease, obesity, osteoporosis and chronic fatigue. DHEA has also been found to help rheumatoid arthritis by relieving pain and morning stiffness. Users have reported being able to reduce their anti-inflammatory medication.

DHEA is on free-sale in the US and can be obtained in the UK from doctors who specialize in Nutritional Medicine. It is also available from some nutritionists. Whilst it is said to be non-toxic, it would be wise to have a saliva test and have the results interpreted by a qualified practitioner before embarking on self-medication. For more information contact Higher Nature (or, for American readers, Aeron Life Cycles) – see Useful Addresses, pages 211 and 218.

One sign that you could be low in this hormone is the loss of hair on the lower third of the legs. Taking supplements of DHEA has benefited many people, but as has been said this should be monitored by a physician.

IBS and Candida Albicans

The parasitic yeast *Candida Albicans* (Thrush) is a fungus which lives on and in our bodies; it is part of our ecosystem. It is normally found in the bowel and mouth from infancy and so long as it stays in those areas, where the body's defence system can keep it under control, all is well. But we are hearing more and more about *Candida* in the popular press. Is it really such a health hazard for some people, or is it just the 'in thing' to have?

The answer is that, unfortunately, chronic candidiasis *is* a serious thing and it does cause health problems, including the Irritable Bowel Syndrome. It could be argued that the problem is not new, but that it has simply gone unnoticed for years. Medical awareness of candidiasis is still poor, but as public awareness grows many people are using self-help methods with good results. Chronic *Candida* can be controlled and full health restored except, perhaps, where it co-exists with a serious illness such as AIDS.

A Man-Made Problem

The increase in fungal infections over the past three decades seems to be the result of ecological carelessness towards the planet and the human body. The pollution of the planet needs no elaboration, but the gradual weakening of the human immune system has not had so much publicity; the damage done there is more subtle, but just as sinister. Many medications – substances which purport to restore or maintain health – start the damage; we complete it by our insistence on fuelling our bodies with a diet which at best is unhelpful, and at worst harmful.

Some of the medicines involved in causing *Candida* are undoubtedly vital in life-threatening illnesses, but the injudicious use of them can also be life-threatening, or at the very least can cause chronic ill-health. These medicines include antibiotics, contraceptive pills, steroids, tranquillizers, sleeping pills in the Valium group, and some ulcer medications.

How Does *Candida* Affect the Bowel?

In the gut, the happy *Candida* live off the fat – or in this case the sugar – of the land, have the dark moist conditions they love; they are aided and abetted by antibiotics, which kill off their enemies the good bacteria. The contraceptive pill and steroids seem to act as fertilizers. Although it is unclear why, it has been observed that when long-term users of tranquillizers and sleeping pills (the benzo-diazepines) are cutting down or stopping their pills, *Candida* problems start. Typically, the most severe problems occur six to twelve months after complete withdrawal. The result is that large numbers of people walk around with a digestive system equal to a gardener's 'grow bag' – a Shangri-La for these nasty little colonizers.

As the *Candida* takes over, the bowel becomes an overactive fermentation tank; a great deal of gas is formed, causing abdominal bloating and often an alteration in bowel habits, diarrhoea or constipation. Is it beginning to sound familiar?

Does it Only Affect the Bowel?

No, it can move around; *Candida* can change from the simple form which causes oral or vaginal thrush to the invasive mycelial fungal form. This more sinister organism grows root-like tendrils which can actually penetrate the wall of its habitat. Instead of being a sealed unit the bowel becomes a leaking pipe through which the waste products of digestion, and the poisons manufactured in the 'Candida chemical factory' can escape into the bloodstream causing widespread problems. The Candida has a perfect transportation system to parts of the body which it does not normally inhabit and where there is no defence system to cope with it. The list of symptoms caused by chronic candidiasis is formidable – extremely long and with many apparently unrelated symptoms:

- *constipation*
- *diarrhoea*
- *bloating*
- *allergies*
- *cystitis*
- *thrush*
- *acne*
- *scaly rashes*
- *nail bed infections*
- *sore tongue*
- *cracks at the side of the mouth*
- *sores in the nose*
- *ear infections*
- *athlete's foot*
- *depression*
- *anxiety*
- *irritability*
- *premenstrual tension*

Can it Affect the Nerves?

Yes it can. Chronic candidiasis is no longer caused by a simple yeast but by a complex organism capable of producing severe physical and psychological illness – psychological illness caused by the waste products of the Candida altering the chemistry of the brain. The resulting symptoms can range from irritability, confusion, and hopelessness to severe anxiety, depression, and a schizophrenia-like illness. Food and chemical allergies are frequently seen in people with chronic *Candida* problems, and because the symptoms include depression and anxiety it is often thought to be psychiatric illness.

Where Does it Cause Trouble?

Infections appear not only at the expected sites – in the mouth, between the toes, on the skin, in the vagina, around the penis and nail-beds – but also throughout the whole of the digestive tract. Sufferers often say, 'I am sore from my mouth to my anus.' So by the time the ears, sinuses, throat and bladder are added, few parts of the body escape. Also, because the forty-plus chemicals produced by the fungus include hormones, the endocrine system can be upset, causing menstrual problems, severe pre-menstrual tension, impotence and thyroid dysfunction. It is important to note that some people with Candida-induced Irritable Bowel Syndrome do not have any other signs of fungal infection such as athlete's foot or thrush.

Candida – What Can Happen at the Doctor's?

Scenario a)

Patient: Doctor, my bowel is worse. I'm so bloated and not sleeping; it's getting me down. There was a bit in a magazine about a fungus in the bowel called *Candida*; could it be that?

Doctor: You worry too much, Mrs Lamb – and don't believe all you read in magazines. No, *Candida* is only a problem in the vagina and in babies' mouths. Have you had any more thoughts about a part-time job?

Scenario b)

Patient: My bowel is getting worse. I had afternoon tea with a friend and I blew up like a balloon. It is always the same if I eat bread or anything sugary. I try to keep off these things but I get such a craving for them. It's like needing a drug. You can see how much weight

I have put on. There was a doctor on the radio saying that sugar craving can be sign of thrush in the bowel; could that be my trouble?

Doctor: Well it's possible. We could try you on an anti-fungal drug for a couple of weeks to see if it helps.

Scenario c)

Patient: Doctor I'm really depressed with this bowel trouble. My diet is becoming very restricted, I am always tired and I have lost a stone in weight. Do you think it could have anything to do with this? (She produces an article on *Candida*).

Doctor: I'm certainly seeing a big increase in fungal infections, so it's a possibility. Let's see, yes, you had antibiotics for that septic toe and you have had three prescriptions for pessaries for thrush this year. It could well be a fungal problem.

Patient: Will I need more tests?

Doctor: There isn't a reliable test for overgrowth of bowel *Candida*.

Patient: Can you send me to a specialist?

Doctor: I'm afraid not; there are very few doctors in the Health Service who deal with problems like this. You could see a clinical nutritionist privately, but it could be costly. The alternative is for me to start you on a course of a drug called Nystatin. It has been around a long time and is quite safe but, to be honest, a lot of people do not tolerate it well. It can kill off the yeast cells too quickly and the poisons from them can make you feel pretty rotten.

Patient: I will gladly put up with being off-colour for a couple of weeks if it will clear this bowel.

Doctor: No, you would have to be on it for several months. I think the best plan would be to see if I can get the pharmacist to order one of the newer anti-fungal substances. They are from plants and seem to work well. You will have to keep to a diet *and* look after yourself a bit more; you try to do too much.

What Happens Next?

Mrs A feels worse; she still has her symptoms and her doctor thinks she is imagining them.

Mr B's self-esteem has not suffered because he *has* been listened to, but unfortunately, two weeks' treatment will not achieve much; also, he is likely to feel much worse at first, and as the reason for this has not been explained he may discontinue treatment. In addition, diet was not mentioned and this is an important part of the treatment.

Mrs C comes out on top; she has the correct information, she has been reassured, she will have continued support, and should do very well.

Killing Off the *Candida*

Note: do not follow these diets if they conflict with instructions from your medical practitioner.

Plan One

The Common-Sense Approach: For People who are Overweight or Normal Weight for their Height and Build.

Your aims:

1   *to cut down the* Candida's *food*
2   *to build up the immune system*

Remember: your loss is also the Candida's loss

CUT OUT OR RESTRICT:
- *Bread: one wholemeal slice daily*
- *All food and drinks containing sugar*
- *All refined cereal products such as white bread, breakfast cereals, biscuits, cakes*
- *Sweets, chocolate, ice cream, soft drinks*

- *Alcohol*
- *Foods containing yeast such as cheese, particularly blue cheese, and vinegar*
- *Citrus fruits or drinks containing citric acid*
- *Any vitamin preparations containing yeast, particularly brewer's yeast.*

(You can use brewer's yeast powder or tablets to help you determine whether or not you have a *Candida* problem. Take it for three or four days and if you have not developed an itchy rectum, bloated or uncomfortable abdomen, diarrhoea, rashes or insomnia, then it is unlikely you have a *Candida* overgrowth.)

EAT:

- *Lots of vegetables, particularly green vegetables, salads and garlic*
- *Fish, meat, poultry*
- *Plain live yoghurt, cottage cheese*
- *Lentils, peas, chick peas, beans, nuts, seeds, buckwheat, and all whole grains*
- *Rice, oats, barley and millet*
- *Peeled fruit (the bloom on the skin of fruit is fungus), limited to two pieces per day*

Why Garlic?

Garlic is a safe, very powerful anti-fungal agent; if you place crushed garlic near a culture of *Candida Albicans*, even the fumes will kill the fungus. If possible take three cloves daily; crush it (it must be crushed to release allicin, the anti-fungal substance) and take it with something like yoghurt or milk and swallow quickly like a medicine. It may burn and make you feel slightly sick but this feeling is soon replaced by a comforting warmth. Wash it down with lots of water. It can also be taken on tomatoes with olive oil, but make sure you eat the whole clove. If you can take three cloves daily it will be devastating for the *Candida* and also lower your cholesterol and blood pressure, detoxify your body and increase your energy and libido. The wonders of garlic are described in *Garlic: The Life-blood of Good Health* by Stephen Fulder (published by Thorsons).

If taking fresh garlic is totally unacceptable to you, your bowel or your friends, you could try a commercial preparation, but ensure that it contains the allicin, as sometimes this is lost in the processing. Kyolic, available in most health stores, is an effective product. One slight drawback to be aware of – garlic can disturb the blood sugar levels and may increase craving for sweet foods. You could try sucking a low-sugar mint, but not too many if you have diarrhoea, as many low-sugar and sugar-free products contain an amino acid called Phenylalanine which if used in excess, can cause diarrhoea. Sorbitol can also have this effect.

TAKE:

- *A good quality, yeast free, multi-mineral and vitamin product*
- *Either lots of live yoghurt or an acidophilus supplement (available by mail order (see page 210) or in most health shops). If you are milk-intolerant make sure the acidophilus has been grown on carrots.*

Remember, if the immune system is strengthened, it can recognize the enemy. The fact that you have *Candida* shows that your immune system is unhappy. Are you looking after its basic needs? Are you getting repeated infections? Does it have to cope with a resident source of infection such as a rotten tooth, infected gums or mucus being swallowed from an infection at the back of the nose?

When you feel well and the *Candida* symptoms have disappeared you can cautiously go back to the diet of your choice, although you will probably find that if you resume a sugar-laden diet your symptoms will reappear.

What Else Can I Do Apart from Diet?

1   *Cut out or reduce the poisons you take daily: smoking, alcohol, caffeine.*
2   *Ask your doctor to review your medications.*
3   *Look after your lymphatic system – exercise.*
4   *Get fresh air, sunlight and daylight.*
5   *Take relaxation seriously.*

Plan Two

All-Out Attack: For People who are Overweight or the Correct Weight for their Build and Height.

This is plan one, plus:

1 A stricter diet
2 Anti-fungal substances
3 Treating food intolerance: food elimination
4 More supplements
5 Treating all other sites of infection

A Stricter Diet

This diet cuts down the amount of carbohydrate in flour or cereal form to about 60 gms (2 ozs). You may feel this is not enough but don't forget all the vegetables and pulses you will be eating will provide more. Little books giving the carbohydrate value of foods can be bought in some supermarkets or newsagents. A rough guide is that a slice of bread from a large loaf is about 30 gms. If you buy any packaged foods study the labels.

FORBIDDEN:

- *Sugar in any form*
- *Bread, biscuits, cakes, cereals*
- *Yeast products: mushrooms, vinegar, pickles, alcohol, marmite*
- *Anything containing citric acid such as tonic water and tinned soup*
- *All dairy products except live yoghurt and cottage cheese; there is a lot of argument about the last two – some doctors allow them, some don't*
- *Fruit and fruit juices for the first month; after that two servings daily (but still no lemons, oranges, grapefruits or limes) of well-washed or peeled fruit, or freshly-squeezed juice.*

RESTRICT:

- *Whole grains: three rice cakes, two oat cakes, two ryvita, one serving of rice, oats or other cereal, daily*

EAT:

- *Potatoes in any form*
- *Mountains of vegetables and salads*
- *Meat, fish, chicken, turkey, duck, rabbit*
- *Eggs*
- *Nuts, seeds, lentils, beans*
- *Olive oil, sunflower oil*

If you try this for a month you may not need to take drugs, but even if you do need to take them it is still a good plan to follow the regime for three to four weeks before you start the drugs. This will help you avoid a condition called *die back* or Herxheimer reaction; if you kill off too much *Candida* at once, the poisons from the dead cells can give you a fever, headache and generally make you feel wretched. This has been noticed most with a drug called Nystatin. The *Candida* is killed by contact with the Nystatin so if possible it is better to use it in powdered form. The tablets available on the NHS do not dissolve until they are in the large bowel so they would miss the *Candida* in the upper digestive tract. If your doctor is willing to prescribe the powder your pharmacist could get further information from the British Society for Nutritional Medicine (see Useful Addresses section). The alternative could be to crush the tablets and put them in water.

Anti-Fungal Substances

Nystatin: your doctor would have to prescribe this. It has been around for many years but to be effective for chronic bowel overgrowth *at least eight weeks' medication is necessary.* If you feel ill when you start taking it (you should not if you have had the strict diet first) take a smaller amount and build up to the full dosage. Many people have noticed that long-term irritating problems such as unpleasant vaginal smells (even when there is no sign of thrush), sore ears, rashes on the face, athlete's foot and sinus troubles also clear up when they have anti-fungal treatment.

Caprylic Acid: This is made from coconuts. It is available in health shops but the slow-release form, *Mycopryl*, can be more effective. You can order it by mail from Biocare, 54 Northfield Road, Kings Norton, Birmingham B30 1JH (0121) 433 3727. They also have a wide range of other products for *Candida*, food allergies and cystitis.

Plan Three

If You Are Underweight.

You really should have professional help but if this is not possible eat as full a diet as possible with plenty of potatoes, whole grains, protein, olive oil and oily fish such as sardines and tuna. Remember if you are relying on sugary foods to maintain your weight you are not only eating empty calories – calories without nutritional benefits – but you are also feeding the *Candida*. The B vitamins can stimulate the appetite but take care with vitamin C. You certainly need plenty but it may have to come from food sources, as vitamin C supplements often reduce the appetite.

How Others Have Coped

Jonathan was healthy as a young child but became 'run down' when he was 7 after the death of his grandfather. For three years he had regular ear and throat infections for which he was prescribed antibiotics. He never felt really well and often complained of tummy aches and diarrhoea.

He had more antibiotics when he was 16. This time it was for acne; he took them for two years. He had never really lost his digestive problems and they began to get worse. His family had always teased him about his 'sweet tooth' but by the time he was 21 he realized how much he craved sweet foods, bread and cheese. He often felt thick-headed or depressed and noticed this was much worse after drinking beer, even half a pint.

When his penis became sore and swollen he was again prescribed antibiotics. This treatment was without effect and was followed by a week on anti-fungal drugs. These helped but the infection recurred when they were stopped. By this time he felt very depressed; walking was so painful he could not get to college. Antibiotics and anti-fungal drugs were tried together and this helped but the infection returned each time the drugs were discontinued.

Jonathan had seen his mother's arthritis improve dramatically when she changed her diet so he decided to see her counsellor. He took the raw garlic suggested and had a half-hearted attempt at the anti-*Candida* diet. His penis was not so sore but he still felt low and it was not until he kept to a strict diet, took nutritional supplements and acidophilus that he really began to improve. He also started to exercise and spend more time outdoors. Within a month the diarrhoea that had been a problem since childhood had gone, he felt much more energetic and his skin was clearer than it had been for years.

Tracy was very tearful when she came for help. She had been off hard drugs for two years and was struggling to get fit; she had also given up smoking and alcohol, but could not understand why she felt so awful. She looked pale and bloated, she lacked energy and felt so irritable just before her period that to avoid company (she had never been violent but feared it was a possibility) she would stay in bed. She had suffered from cystitis twice and thrush three times in the preceding six months. She had a lot of dandruff; there was a scaly red rash around her hairline. She went on to a strict anti-*Candida* programme and gave up tea. She used Selsun (anti-fungal) shampoo and had two short sessions on a sunbed weekly. This cleared the rash on her face. Her room-mate complained loudly about the smell of garlic so she changed to Kyolic (page 79). At the end of the first week change was visible; she was not so bloated and said she was not bursting into tears all the time. After the third week she had lost several pounds in weight and was glowing with health.

Bowel Infections

Many people with the Irritable Bowel Syndrome can date it from a bowel infection, often after a trip abroad, after flu or a cold where they have swallowed a lot of mucus or any condition where they have been given antibiotics.

Parasites

It is commonly supposed that infestation with parasites is only a problem in tropical countries; in fact it is a source of bowel problems in Europe, America and Australia. Infection with protozoa (single-celled organisms) *Giardia lambia* and *Entamoeba histolytica* can be spread through water, food and pets. It multiplies rapidly, causes a watery diarrhoea with bloating, abdominal pain and exhaustion. Medical help is necessary for this condition which can be diagnosed by investigation of the stool, or mucus from the wall of the rectum. There are drugs for this condition but the herb *Artemia annua* has been found to be very effective. Raw garlic also kills parasites. If parasite infections are neglected they can cause chronic ill-health. Irritable Bowel Syndrome and food intolerance can often be traced back to *Giardia* infestation.

Spreading the Word

The work of two American doctors, C. Orion Truss and William G. Crook, has been valuable in alerting both professionals and the public to the *Candida* problem, but how long will it be before their pioneering efforts are universally accepted? Until 'Candida-consciousness' is raised, not only are sufferers from the more severe mental and physical manifestations of chronic candidiasis going to be misdiagnosed and inappropriately treated, but also sufferers from infections (for example, of the bladder, ears, and skin) thought to be bacterial in origin, are going to have their conditions aggravated by antibiotics and steroids.

For further reading on this subject:

Candida Albicans: Could Yeast be your Problem by Leon Chaitow, Thorsons.
The Yeast Connection by William G. Crook, Biosocial Publications, Europe.
The Missing Diagnosis by C. Orion Truss, P.O. Box 26508, Birmingham AL 35226 U.S.A.
Coping with Anxiety and Depression by Shirley Trickett, Sheldon Press.

12

IBS and M.E.
(Myalgic Encephalomyelitis)

M.E. (Myalgic Encephalomyelitis), Malingerer's Disease or Royal Free Disease

People with M.E. are often diagnosed as having the Irritable Bowel Syndrome – which in effect they have and need to be treated for – but they also need help with other problems. M.E. is a chronic illness which produces bouts of extreme tiredness in the muscles and brain. It can start with an illness like glandular fever or flu; sometimes it is so severe people have to give up work for a time. Sufferers from this condition have been classed as malingerers or hypochondriacs for decades. M.E. was first recorded about fifty years ago, but it has only been in the past few years that there has been a sharing of information among sufferers and doctors. M.E. is often mistaken for nervous illness because the symptoms include anxiety, depression and lethargy. The immune system is also affected and multiple allergies and *Candida* can be present.

Research into M.E. is being carried out at St Mary's Hospital, London and elsewhere, but as yet, there are few answers in conventional medicine. However the approach of some complementary therapies has helped many people to recover completely. The important aspects of treatment are rest, a healthy diet, supplements, fresh air, daylight, and keeping the bowel as clean as possible by preventing constipation, restoring the normal balance to the gut bacteria. Any therapy which promotes relaxation and natural healing is also recommended. Tranquillizers rarely help this condition, they merely add more poisons to a body already struggling hard to excrete the poisons caused by the virus. Sometimes a night-time dose of a sedative anti-depressant is helpful where insomnia is severe and where normal sleep-wake cycles are trying to be established.

Important Point: While there are several exercise suggestions for stimulating the immune system in this book, they are not appropriate for people with M.E. because the muscles are affected. For these people rest is the priority.

The Homoeopathic Hospital in London takes GP referrals for M.E.

For further information write to:

M.E. Association,
P.O. Box 8
Stanford Le Hope,
Essex SS17 8EX (Enclosing SAE)

M.E. Action Campaign
Mr Martin Lev
P.O. Box 1126
London W3 0RY

Reading on M.E.

M.E. *Post Vital Fatigue Syndrome* by Dr Anne Macintyre (Thorsons, 1998)
M.E. *What Is It – Have You Got It? – How to Get Better* by Mike Franklin and Jane Sullivan (Random Century, 1989)

Radionically prepared homoeopathic remedies for M.E. (*Aprevir*)
and *Candida (Candirad)* are available from Mrs D. Frankish
M.Rad.a., 4 Relton Terrace, Monkseaton, Whitley Bay,
Tyne and Wear NE25 8DY.

13

IBS and Food Intolerance

We are all familiar with stories of severe allergic reactions where a person reacts violently to one food and has to avoid it for life; we hear people say: 'I dare not eat fish/strawberries/peanuts/eggs because my mouth swells up, my eyes itch and I have trouble breathing.' This condition is widely recognized by the medical profession and it is accepted that prompt medical intervention is often necessary. The condition that is less well known and accepted medically is that of food intolerance.

What Happens in Food Intolerance?

The toxic colon and *Candida* have already been discussed. Because of these and other conditions including damage from drugs and pollution, it seems our digestive systems are becoming less efficient. Because of this, larger molecules of undigested food are allowed to pass into the bloodstream. The immune system attacks them because they are unfamiliar and the result can be trouble in any part of the body. The symptoms are not dramatic and easily recognized, as in food allergy, but there can be a confusion of odd symptoms which may mimic numerous other conditions such as asthma or arthritis. After years of this problem the sufferer can have severe weight loss and be completely exhausted. Milder symptoms include:

- *bloating*
- *flushing*
- *palpitations*
- *headache*
- *anxiety or depression after eating the offending foods.*

The condition responds well to treatment, but because of the lack of information it can be difficult to find someone who understands the problem. Some clinical nutritionists believe many chronic conditions, such as certain chest and kidney troubles and arthritis, are caused by food intolerance. The dramatic improvement in some degenerative and nervous illnesses in people who have been treated for food intolerance – even if they have only used self-help methods – would seem to confirm this. Here is Margaret's story:

It all started when I was pregnant. I had lost a lot of weight and my bowel movement was never normal; I either had diarrhoea or constipation. After my son was born I had a rash on my legs which formed blisters.

The doctor said it was post-natal depression and gave me tranquillizers. This went on for years, I was convinced it was something to do with food but I was given more and more tranquillizers, then anti-depressants. When I developed migraine – although it seemed like the last straw – it put me on the right road. I found a book in the health shop on headaches. It was the first time I had heard of food intolerance or elimination diets. I cut out all dairy produce, chocolate, tea and coffee and did improve a little but it was not until I had an asthma attack after drinking a glass of orange squash (containing E102, Tartrazine) that the doctor began to think about allergies. He referred me to a private doctor who just said I had severe allergies and sent me to a dietician. This was not very helpful and it was not until I found a doctor with an interest in clinical nutrition that I started to make progress. Tests revealed I had trouble with wheat, yeast and several other foods. The treatment suggested was an elimination/anti-*Candida* diet, vitamins and minerals.

I really feel I am getting somewhere; for the first time in years my head is clear, I am not depressed, and my silly bowel is starting to behave.

Several Foods Affect Me – What Can I Do?

If you cannot find a doctor who understands the problem you will have to rely on self-help. You could start with the common-sense approach first:

1 *Clean out your digestive tract.*
2 *Avoid the foods you know upset you plus all the common allergens: wheat, dairy products, citrus fruits, eggs and additives.*
3 *Strengthen your immune system with exercise, relaxation, sunlight (or daylight), fresh air and vitamin and mineral supplements.*

Food Rotation

Some people react to so many foods that they could not possibly exclude them all because they would become malnourished. The answer is to eat most things but only once in four days. The body seems to be able to cope with this and many people do well on rotation diets. It is of course tedious, as all these diets are; it would involve eating everything to do with the cow – dairy produce and beef – on one day, and everything connected with sheep – lamb, lamb's liver, ewe's milk yoghurt – on another day, and so on; also a different grain, vegetable and fruit every fourth day. There are many books around which describe food intolerance in detail and offer a variety of exclusion diets, good choices would be *Food Allergy and Intolerance* by Jonathan Brostoff and Linda Gamlin, Bloomsbury, *Perhaps It's An Allergy* by Ellen Rothera, Food & Chemical Allergy Association, or *The Food Allergy Plan* by Keith Mumby, Unwin.

Chemical Intolerance

Offending substances don't always gain access to the body through the mouth; they can be inhaled or absorbed through the skin. Bearing this in mind perhaps it is time to consider what chemicals you are spraying on your head, under your arms, up your nose and on your skin. Use simple non-perfumed toilet preparations and don't buy aerosol cans. You could try pure essential oils in the bath; many of them smell wonderful. They may not affect you the way synthetic perfumes do.

It is time also to throw out all the household cleaning agents and get back to simple soaps (non-biological washing powders) and old-fashioned wax furniture polish. The wood likes it better too. There is a whole range of ecological domestic cleaning products. The washing-up liquid has been particularly helpful for many people; a tight chest while washing up is very common in people with chemical allergies. A simple product called Chemico, a pink paste made from powdered rock which has been manufactured in Britain for about seventy years is gentle and safe and cleans everything, sinks, cookers, floors, even windows. It is very cheap here but is now being sold in America at $12 per tin!

Allergy Switch Off, a safe product for symptomatic relief, is available from The Sanford Clinic, 15 Lake Road North, Roath Park, Cardiff CF2 5QA (01222) 747507.

14

IBS and Prescribed Drugs

Antibiotics

After reading the *Candida* chapter you will not be surprised that there are complaints of long-term digestive upsets from people who have taken antibiotics. If you have an infection that has failed to respond to natural healing methods such as garlic, fluids and rest, you may need to take an antibiotic. You can minimize trouble by replacing the good bacteria in the bowel which are being killed off by the drug by eating live yoghurt or finding a supplement in your health store which contains *Lactobacillus acidophilus* (see page 79). If you have been on antibiotics long-term you may also need to take a yeast-free vitamin B complex formula.

CAUTION:

1 *You may risk severe illness if you have a serious infection and refuse antibiotics.*
2 *You may now be allergic to an antibiotic you were formerly able to tolerate.*

Tranquillizers and Sleeping Pills

The effect of tranquillizers and sleeping pills on the gut is unclear, but there is no doubt that a very high percentage of users develop the Irritable Bowel Syndrome and chronic candidiasis either during therapy or during withdrawal. The symptoms can persist for many years after complete withdrawal from the drugs.

More gastro-intestinal problems were reported in people taking lorazepam (Ativan) than other drugs in the same group, such as diazepam (Valium). It is known that these drugs block the absorption of zinc so it is possible that they hinder the absorption of other vital nutrients, thus allowing the body to become depleted; *Candida* thrives in these circumstances. Here are some typical experiences:

June had been off diazepam (Valium) for two years. The first six months had been very rough but she coped well and was pleased with her progress. She had much more energy and felt she was coming alive again; the depression she had experienced for years had gone. When she had been drug-free for about ten months she started to have digestive troubles – constipation, bloating and pain. She was fully investigated at the hospital and told she had the Irritable Bowel Syndrome. The high-fibre diet made her symptoms worse, everything she ate seemed to upset her, the skin around her anus itched and became sore and her ears itched and discharged a watery fluid. When this touched her face it caused a rash. Altogether she was very low and could not understand what was happening to her. When she saw a television programme about tranquillizer withdrawal she rang the counselling line and things began to fall into place. They recommended a book and in it she read about the *Candida* connection and the large numbers of people who have been on these drugs and then experienced bowel problems.

At her local health food shop she found a book on *Candida* and she bought the supplements it recommended. She was unable to tolerate these in the suggested doses so she started with a small dose and gradually increased it. A relative paid for her to have a week at a health farm and she felt this helped her a great deal. She was given an 80 per cent raw diet and was astonished to find that many of the vegetables she could not digest when they were cooked proved no trouble when they were raw. (This is quite a common experience.) She continued with the diet at home and tried to take more care of her general health. She washed her hair frequently with an anti-fungal shampoo and used an anti-fungal nappy rash cream on her face. She felt much better after a few weeks and felt well six months later although she did notice if she strayed too far from the anti-*Candida* diet her bowel symptoms returned.

Martin was down to ½ mg of lorazepam (Ativan) when his bowel troubles started. He complained of abdominal pain, and bloating, and his bowel movements were erratic: sometimes he was constipated then he would have a loose stool for several days. He had investigations which showed nothing abnormal. He noticed his bladder felt sore after drinking orange juice or beer and he found several foods he had always enjoyed now upset him. He was not convinced about the *Candida* connection at first but after speaking with people who had come off tranquillizers and had the same problem he decided to ask his GP for a course of Nystatin. His doctor had supported several people through withdrawal and was very helpful. He prescribed an eight-week course of Nystatin. After the first week he began to feel better, he was not so bloated and was sleeping better. He gave up dairy produce and kept to a low carbohydrate diet and small regular meals. Athlete's foot had plagued him for months; this also cleared up.

Joyce had been off her sleeping pills (temazepam) for eighteen months. During the early months she had suffered a lot of sleepless nights but had coped well. When she rang a tranquillizer support line she was embarrassed by how distressed she was, but as she explained, she felt she had gone back to square one, and was feeling as ill as she had in early withdrawal. To make matters worse she had some strange symptoms and her husband said she was being silly: she felt sick and dizzy when she was near strong perfumes; cleaning products she had always used made her feel ill. She had always enjoyed shopping but she now found she felt headachy and sick in certain department stores. She had suffered panic attacks in early withdrawal and knew these feelings were different. Eating was also a problem; her pulse raced and she had hot flushes after certain foods. It was such an odd collection of symptoms she wondered if she was imagining them and was greatly reassured when she was told about *Candida* and food and chemical intolerance. Because she had lost a lot of weight and was by now confused about which foods upset her, she decided to see a clinical nutritionist. Here she had a cytotoxic test (a sample of blood is looked at under the microscope after it has been in contact with various foods to see whether the white blood cells react or not), and was then given an exclusion diet and supplements. The first three weeks were a struggle and she did not feel she was getting very far, then she started to feel stronger and gained two pounds in weight. Six months later she felt well and was working full time.

While the post-withdrawal problems of tranquillizer use are not yet widely medically accepted, particularly with regard to *Candida* and food intolerance, the dangers of long-term use of these drugs are well known.

Reading for Professionals

Committee on Safety of Medicines: Current Problems, Number 21, January 1988.

Benzodiazepines

Dependence and withdrawal symptoms: there has been concern for many years regarding benzodiazepine dependence (*Br.Med.J.* 1980: 280, 910–912). Such dependence is becoming increasingly worrying. Withdrawal symptoms include anxiety, tremor, confusion, insomnia, perception disorders, fits, depression, gastrointestinal and other somatic symptoms. These may sometimes be difficult to distinguish from the symptoms of the original illness.

It is important to note that withdrawal symptoms can occur with benzodiazepines following therapeutic doses given for short periods of time. Withdrawal effects usually appear shortly after stopping a benzodiazepine with a short half-life. Symptoms may continue for weeks or months. No epidemiological evidence is available to suggest that one benzodiazepine is more responsible for the development of dependency or withdrawal symptoms than another. The Committee on Safety of Medicines recommends that the use of benzodiazepines should be limited in the following ways:

As anxiolytics

1 *Benzodiazepines are indicated for the short-term relief (two to four weeks only) of anxiety that is severe, disabling or subjecting the individual to unacceptable distress, occurring alone or in association with insomnia or short-term psychosomatic organic or psychotic illness.*

2 *The use of benzodiazepines to treat short-term 'mild' anxiety is inappropriate and unsuitable.*

As hypnotics [Sleep inducing drugs]

1 *Benzodiazepines should be used to treat insomnia only when it is severe, disabling, or subjecting the individual to extreme distress.*

Dose

1 *The lowest dose which can control the symptoms should be used. It should not be continued beyond four weeks.*

2 *Long-term chronic use is not recommended.*

3 *Treatment should always be tapered off gradually.*

4 *Patients who have taken benzodiazepines for a long time may require a longer period during which doses are reduced.*

5 *When a benzodiazepine is used as a hypnotic, treatment should, if possible, be intermittent.*

Precautions

1 *Benzodiazepines should not be used alone to treat depression or anxiety associated with depression. Suicide may be precipitated in such patients.*

2 *They should not be used for phobic or obsessional states.*

3 *They should not be used for the treatment of chronic psychosis.*

4   In case of loss or bereavement, psychological adjustment may be inhibited by benzodiazepines.

5   Disinhibiting effects may be manifested in various ways. Suicide may be precipitated in patients who are depressed, and aggressive behaviour towards self and others may be precipitated. Extreme caution should therefore be used in prescribing benzodiazepines in patients with personality disorders.

Complete List of Benzodiazepines

Only those marked with an asterisk (*) are now available on the NHS.

Medical Name	Brand Name(s)
Alprazolam	Xapax
Bromazepam	Lexotan
Chlordiazepoxide*	Librium, Tropium
Clobazam*	Frisium
Clorazepate potassium	Tranxene
Diazepam*	Valium, Alupram, Atensine, Evacalm, Solis, Tensium
Flunitrazepam	Rohypnol
Flurazepam	Dalmane
Ketazolam	Anxon
Loprazolam	Dormonoct
Lorazepam*	Ativan, Almazine
Lormetazepam	Noctamid
Medazepam	Nobrium
Nitrazepam*	Mogadon, Nitrados, Noctesed Remnos, Somnite
Oxazepam*	Serenid-D
Prazepam	Centrax
Temazepam*	Normison
Triazolam*	Halcion

Caution: these drugs have been known to cause dependence; consult your doctor, withdraw slowly, and read Coming off Tranquilizers and Sleeping Pills by Shirley Trickett, Thorsons.

Tagamet, Zantac (Cimetidine, Ranitidine)

These drugs have been a breakthrough in the treatment of gastric ulcers and have saved countless people from the surgeon's knife. It would seem, however, that because the drugs have been around for some time, because they are useful, and because they do not seem to have any serious side-effects, a complacency towards them has developed. People are being left on them far too long, month after month, year after year, without any review. A conscientious medical practitioner would be shocked by this, but this is the reality of the situation. It is not surprising, therefore, that there are increasing calls about this group of drugs.

The odd thing is that while these drugs seem effective in the treatment of ulcers, some people complain of developing bowel problems during therapy. Here is *Olivia's* story:

Five years ago I was prescribed Tagamet and a bland diet for a suspected ulcer. This improved and after a few months I returned to a normal diet. I began to have very painful bowel movements and felt uncomfortable and bloated. The doctor diagnosed the Irritable Bowel Syndrome. I was issued repeat prescriptions for Tagamet and after two years decided I should stop taking it; I felt dreadful, anxious, irritable and depressed. After a couple of weeks I felt so ill I was glad to start taking it again; the symptoms vanished. Two years later I decided I must come off no matter how I felt. Months of headaches, anxiety and depression followed, but the bowel symptoms disappeared. For the first time in years I have a pain-free, normal bowel movement.

Caution:

1 *These drugs increase the potency of tranquillizers and sleeping pills.*
2 *Anecdotal evidence (in the United Kingdom and the United States) suggests that they can cause dependence; withdrawal reactions have been reported.*
3 *Post-withdrawal fungal infections have been reported.*
4 *Bowel problems during Cimetidine therapy have been reported.*

Can Other Prescribed Drugs Cause Bowel Problems?

Yes they can – arthritis, drugs, steroids, water tablets, beta blockers to name a few. Check with your doctor that the medication you are taking is necessary and if it is, take care to keep the bowel as clean as possible and take supplements or live yoghurt to encourage the growth of helpful bacteria.

Caution: do not stop taking any medication without consulting your doctor.

Street Drugs

All hard drugs cause absorption problems and in addition users often have little appetite. Ideally a good diet and supplements should start several weeks before detoxification begins. Bowel problems and *Candida* are frequently seen after withdrawal from hard drugs.

PART
TWO

Self-Help
Methods

15

IBS and Negative Emotions

Negative emotions can affect the harmony of the digestive system – anger, prolonged grief, frustration, anxiety and depression all take their toll.

Extreme fear can cause the bowel to evacuate spontaneously. A lesser form of this is the constant worrier who always has diarrhoea.

Tension

People who continually suppress their emotions with tension are more likely to be constipated. They might experience tension headaches or pain in the neck and shoulders, but not associate their constipation with tension. When there is an inability to relax, the abdominal muscles can be affected with the result that a person cannot 'let go' of the stool.

Anger

If you are continually angry you certainly risk digestive problems, and not only these but also high blood pressure and heart disease.

Can you imagine an angry person enjoying and fully digesting a hearty meal? Unlikely, I think.

You might justifiably be angry about the situation you have to cope with, but need to ask yourself what purpose is it serving. You are only hurting yourself and probably others around you. Consider whether you are really angry with yourself because of your inability to deal with the situation. If you cannot resolve the situation by honest, open communication with the person or persons who are upsetting you, perhaps it is time to seek counselling. If the relationships in your life are under threat then it is certainly time to take your anger seriously.

Often an angry partner comes home seething with problems from the workplace and vents this on his or her partner who, in turn, becomes angry or irritable with the children. Children, no matter how young, are thinking, feeling human beings who only want to be loved and to love. They are very sensitive to atmosphere. Like little sponges they absorb the tension around them and often blame themselves for being 'naughty'. They can become very fearful. Parents often see this as being difficult and cannot see that they are the cause of the bedwetting, tantrums, failure to keep up at school, the nightmares, disturbed sleep, withdrawal, wanting to spend time in friends' homes rather than their own. Older children might become truculent, play truant or turn to drugs or drink. Some children will start to bully younger children in the home or at school.

The repercussions from one person's anger are frightening. Misplaced anger is a form of bullying. If children are seeing this at home it is not surprising that they react in this way.

If you are in a position of authority and display anger towards your staff, think hard about how many lives you could be affecting.

Prolonged Grief

Grief is a process to be worked through. It has a beginning, a middle and an end. That is not to say that you will ever forget the person you have lost or stop loving them, but if you hang on to grief for years and use it as an excuse to give up on life or to become overdependent on others then it becomes unhealthy. It might indicate that in focusing on loss and sadness you are denying that you are also fearful, angry or feeling guilt. Ask yourself if the person who has gone would be unhappy to see you with constant digestive upsets and only half-living. The national organization Cruise (directory enquiries or the Yellow Pages will give you the number for your area) specializes in bereavement counselling.

Grief often turns into clinical depression. See your doctor. In the short term, antidepressant medication can be of great help to get you back to a more normal life.

Frustration

The effects of this can be similar to anger. The tension produced upsets the digestion, sleeping patterns and mood. It is useless to treat the bowel and take supplements if you are unwilling to face the cause of your frustration. If the cause is not one that you can turn your back on or tackle with real communication (no matter how scary that might be), then seek counselling for help in adapting to the circumstances before your health, the health of those around you and your relationships with people worsen.

Jealousy

People who have not suffered from this distressing emotion or have been on the receiving end of it often see it as a brief twinge of envy. It can be a great deal more serious than that. It can be a threat to physical and mental health, a common reason for the breakdown of relationships and even a cause of violence. It often comes from deep feelings of insecurity and low self-worth. If this emotion is affecting your life see your doctor and ask for referral to a psychologist for long-term counselling. Do not be ashamed or think this is a trivial reason to seek help. It is not a moral issue. A person would not choose to experience this emotion. It is not your fault but you do have a duty to yourself (your health and happiness are important too) and to those around you to learn how to cope with this.

Guilt

This is about the most useless of the negative emotions. What purpose does it serve?

If you have done something you are ashamed of, then the guilt you are feeling has already told you not to repeat that action. You have had your lesson. Why go on punishing yourself? Asking forgiveness of the person or persons concerned and truly forgiving yourself can bring great healing. *Caution:* Only do this if you are sure that purging yourself will not bring distress to anyone. Be open and honest only if it is safe. Seek counselling if this useless emotion is affecting your physical or mental health or ruining relationships.

Some people find it helpful to see a priest for confession and absolution. If you can't bring yourself to do this, perhaps you could take a quiet few minutes to voice your transgression out loud and ask God, the Universe, or however you see the Infinite and ask for forgiveness. Above all, love and forgive yourself.

16

IBS and Hyperventilation

The impression that patients suffering from the Irritable Bowel Syndrome hyperventilated was researched in a three-month study at St Peter's Hospital, Chertsey. It did not prove that there was an association but it was convincing enough to suggest that further study would be worthwhile. Increased swallowing was noted in Irritable Bowel sufferers; this was thought to be the result of hyperventilation making the mouth dry. It also suggested that some symptoms of Irritable Bowel Syndrome may respond well to breathing exercises.

L.C. Lum, formerly Consultant Chest Physician at Papworth Hospital, Cambridge, in his paper 'Hyperventilation Syndromes in Medicine and Psychiatry', (*Journal of the Royal Society of Medicine,* Vol. 80, April 1987, page 119) states that people who hyperventilate frequently have the Irritable Bowel Syndrome, and many have definite symptoms of food intolerance. He also said that many people with food intolerance also have symptoms of hyperventilation.

These findings are not surprising. You will see in this chapter how breathing affects the nerves and anything which upsets the nervous system must have repercussions in the gut. We have also seen how food and chemical intolerance can make the nasal mucosa swell; this in itself is a cause of hyperventilation.

What is Hyperventilation?

Hyperventilation – or overbreathing – is breathing in a rapid, shallow way using the upper chest instead of the abdomen. Breathing in this manner produces more oxygen than the body needs, and the result is a fall in the level of carbon dioxide in the blood. The acid/alkaline balance of the body is also disturbed and this can cause a lot of strange and sometimes frightening feelings. It can result in panic attacks, unreal feelings, headaches, tingling around the mouth and in the feet and hands, a tight chest, pain in the neck and shoulders and digestive upsets.

Here is how it is described in the *Oxford Book of Psychiatry* (1983); it shows how poor breathing habits can affect the whole body.

> Over-breathing is breathing in a rapid and shallow way which results in a fall in the concentration of carbon dioxide in the blood. The resultant symptoms include dizziness, faintness, numbness and tingling in the hands, feet and face, carpopedal spasms (severe cramp in hands and feet), and precordial discomfort (discomfort in the area of the chest over the heart). There is also a feeling of breathlessness which may prolong the condition. When a patient has unexplained bodily symptoms, the possibility of persistent overbreathing should always be borne in mind.

It does not matter what causes hyperventilation; it may be a bloated abdomen cramping your lungs, or a blocked nose that starts the habit, or it may be that you have always been anxious and have been a poor breather since childhood, but no matter what the cause is, the worst symptom of hyperventilation is panic attacks.

Panic Attacks

The sufferer is suddenly overwhelmed by fear for no apparent reason, and often feels that death is not far away. Some people feel unable to move or speak, others shout out for help. Although the attacks usually last only a few minutes it can seem much longer to the sufferer.

In a person who is not nervously ill, an examination or an exciting social event may produce 'butterflies in the stomach', sweating hands, constriction of the chest, a rise in the heart rate and so on – all the feelings of raised adrenalin levels. This is a normal response. A panic attack is an exaggeration of this – the cause is an exhausted nervous system. If you are over-enthusiastic the first time you go out jogging, the next day your muscles will complain by being stiff and sore. Panic attacks, agoraphobia, irritability, and many other symptoms are a similar cry for help from your nervous system; it is saying 'Do not abuse me, I have had enough.'

It is often hard to convince someone who is having panic attacks that it is not the onset of some terrible disease. Every symptom – wildly beating heart, rapid breathing, sweating, shaking – is part of the 'fight or flight' response. We do not want to stop this mechanism because we would not survive long without it, but we do want it to stop over-reacting with full-blown panic at every little stimulation.

If you suffer from this distressing problem and think you have some dreaded disease the following definition, from 'Hyperventilation (shallow breathing) as a Cause of Panic Attacks', Dr Hibbert (British Medical Journal, vol 288, January 1984), should reassure you:

> The syndrome (collection of symptoms) characterised by repeated panic attacks has been known by several names, including muscular exhaustion of the heart, neurasthenia (nervous exhaustion), irritable heart, anxiety neurosis, effort syndrome, and cardiac neurosis. The manual's definition of panic disorder states that attacks are manifested by the sudden onset of intense apprehension, fear or terror, often associated with feelings of impending doom. The most common symptoms experienced during an attack are dyspnoea (breathing

difficulty), choking or smothering sensations, dizziness, vertigo, or unsteady feelings, feelings of unreality, paraesthesias (disordered sensations such as tingling and pins and needles) hot and cold flushes, sweating, faintness, trembling or shaking, and fear of dying, going crazy or doing something uncontrolled during the attack. Attacks usually last minutes; more rarely hours.

How Can I Get Off the Fear Roundabout?

If you try to fight the panic and give yourself messages like, 'I am going to be sick, pass out or wet myself' each time you have a panic attack, you are planting a seed in your mind that will make you react in the same way the next time. It will be the trigger for stimulating more adrenalin, more fear. If on the other hand you teach your body to give the correct messages to your brain, you can break this chain reaction. It is not suggested that it is easy to accomplish and it is not always possible to think clearly enough about what to do when you are actually in the throes of an attack. This is why it is so important to *practise* your response when you are relaxed and give yourself the firm command: 'This is panic and I can control it.'

First Aid for Panic Attacks

Since the main cause of the unpleasant feeling is an imbalance of oxygen and carbon dioxide the aim is to stabilize this as quickly as possible. Let your breath out in a long sigh and then cupping your hands around your mouth. This enables you to re-breathe your own carbon dioxide (don't hold your breath). If you are home you could place a paper – never plastic – bag around your nose and mouth. Do not *blow* or breathe deeply into the bag, just let the breaths come; they will slow down naturally as you get your own carbon dioxide back from the air in the bag. You can also slow the breathing down by splashing cold water on the face or by putting cold cloths or ice packs over the cheeks and nose. A packet of frozen peas wrapped in a dish towel has often been used to good effect.

If breathing is the first thought during panic the second thought should be: '*Eat or drink something sweet as soon as possible*'. Chapter 17 explains why this helps and how eating sugar is only a first-aid measure for panic and should be followed by a meal and a rest.

Become Aware of Your Breathing

It may be several weeks before your breathing habits improve, so be patient with yourself. You might find the following exercises tedious but, as you know, getting better requires effort. (If it does not stop you concentrating on the exercises you could have the radio on.) If your heart is bumping away as you lie down you could try closing your eyes and pressing gently on the eyeballs; this causes a reflex slowing of the heart and can be soothing.

If you pull in your abdomen as you breathe in this restricts the air intake. The aim is to breathe slowly, lifting the abdomen. If you breathe deeply you can become light-headed or your heart may bump a little. This shows how it is not only low carbon dioxide levels, but also rapid changes in those levels, which can cause symptoms. This is nothing to worry about, and if you get in a muddle take a rest and start again.

How Do I Know if I Am Overbreathing?

It is easy to recognize severe hyperventilation: erratic, noisy, rapid breaths where the chest is heaving and the abdomen is barely moving. The person feels the need to take an occasional deep breath and often finds it difficult to breathe out. Hyperventilators sigh a lot.

Chronic overbreathing is not so easy to identify because there is nothing dramatic to see or hear – quiet, shallow rapid breaths with most of the movement from the upper chest.

Breathing Exercises

Make the time to do two half-hour sessions daily. If you are having severe symptoms, panic or agoraphobia, a quick five minutes here and there is not enough. The best times are after breakfast and before the evening meal. Sit comfortably in the chair or, better still, lie on the floor or bed, and loosen tight clothing. As you become more skilled, you will be able to practise abdominal breathing anywhere, even standing in a queue.

Slowly and Gently, *Not* Deeply and Vigorously.

1   *Place one hand on your abdomen and one on your chest. The hand on your chest should stay as still as possible. The hand on your abdomen should go up and down as you breathe; visualize a blue and white boat gently rising and falling in the waves.*
2   *Breathe out through your nose (don't force it), and let your abdomen fall gently as you do so.*
3   *Breathe in through the nose letting the abdomen rise; make the out breath longer than the in breath.*
4   *Gradually train yourself to breathe between eight and twelve times per minute. (Sometime when you are resting, look at a watch with a second hand and count how many times your chest goes up and down (this is one breath) during half a minute; double it and you will have the rate at which you breathe per minute.)*

For more information on panic attacks read *Coping Successfully with Panic Attacks* written by this author and published by Sheldon Press.

17

Low Blood Sugar

At first sight this condition might seem a rather unlikely cause of the Irritable Bowel Syndrome, but if it is considered that low blood sugar levels (and also hyperventilation) are extremely common causes of nervous tension and panic attacks, then the connection cannot be overlooked.

What is it?

Hypoglycaemia or low blood sugar is an abnormally low level of glucose in the blood. The food we eat is turned into glucose by the digestive system and we use the energy it produces to nourish our bodies, rather like putting petrol in a car. If the spaces between meals are too long or the food taken is not sustaining enough, as soon as the stomach is empty, a frantic message goes to the brain saying: 'Help I'm empty, do something.' The brain responds by saying: 'Instructions understood, I'll send a messenger to open the larder door.' The chemical messenger is *adrenalin* and the larder is the *liver*, where a substance like sugar is stored. When the key is turned, the sugar enters the blood stream and raises the blood sugar levels and the symptoms subside. What you must remember is that this takes time, and while this is going on, the sufferer could have experienced a range of unpleasant feelings from being shaky, tired, irritable and having blurred vision or feelings of unreality, to a full-blown panic attack and feelings of despair and deep depression. People who treat their bodies like this day in and day out, risk nervous breakdowns and chronic physical illnesses. Typically they are the people who eat little or no breakfast, have a small lunch and eat a main meal in the evening. They often feel droopy mid-morning or mid-afternoon when they might crave sugar, then they feel sleepy within an hour of the evening meal. Strangely enough, eating little all day does not keep them thin, they are often overweight. The effect of adrenalin on the bowel has been discussed on pages 62–67.

Sugar is Not the Cure

An amazing number of people come saying, 'My doctor says I have low blood sugar and need to take frequent drinks with sugar.' This chapter will show that in fact the opposite is true and that taking sugar makes the symptoms worse by making the pancreas work even harder. Hypoglycaemia could be said to be the opposite to diabetes. In diabetes the pancreas fails to produce the chemical called insulin which enables us to burn the food we eat to produce energy. In hypoglycaemia the situation is the reverse; the pancreas is over-stimulated, usually because of nervous exhaustion, and produces too much insulin. This causes the food we eat to be burned up too quickly and we cannot maintain the levels of blood glucose necessary to function normally.

The results are unpleasant physical effects such as a rapid heart-beat and feeling faint; because the brain cannot store glucose there are also unpleasant brain effects such as anxiety, depression, panic attacks and neurotic behaviour. If you eat sugary foods, particularly when you are very hungry, the pancreas – which is already jittery and in top gear – pushes out more insulin than is necessary to cope with the sugar. The result is a rapid drop in blood sugar levels, and as we have seen the result is a flood of adrenalin.

Familial History

It is very important for people who are from families where there are other low blood sugar problems (asthma, arthritis, allergy and so on) to follow the hypoglycaemic eating plan. It is also wise to start the diet three or four weeks *before* you intend to stop smoking, drinking or before you cut down on tranquillizers or sleeping pills.

Eating Plan to Keep Blood Sugar Levels Stable

If your doctor has already given you a diet to follow consult him or her before you make any changes in your eating pattern. If there are some foods here which you cannot tolerate, just exclude them and follow the main theme.

Principles of the Diet

The aim is to avoid foods and substances that are quickly absorbed in order to minimize rapid changes in the level of glucose in the blood.

Avoid or cut down to a minimum refined carbohydrates:
- *Sugar, sweets, chocolate*
- *White bread, white flour, cakes, biscuits, pastry*
- *Alcohol*
- *Sweet drinks*
- *Junk foods.*

Eat non-refined carbohydrates:
- *Whole grain cereals; wheat, oats, barley, rice, rye, millet.*

Give up processed breakfast cereals and make your own muesli from whole oats, nuts, seeds (sunflower, pumpkin or sesame are all very nutritious) and a little dried fruit (sultanas, apricots etc). If you are used to eating 'plastic bread' you will love the taste of whole-grain brown bread. If you normally eat brown bread make sure it is whole grain.

Eat protein:
- *Animal protein: meat, fish, poultry, cheese, eggs, milk, yoghurt.*
- *Vegetable protein: nuts, seeds, peas, beans, lentils and small amounts in all vegetables.*

There is always a lot of argument about how much protein should be included in any diet. The early diets for low blood sugar were very high in protein. Eating this way certainly controls the blood sugar but more recent research has shown that the body does not like too much concentrated protein, and blood sugar levels can be kept steady on smaller amounts, particularly if lots of raw vegetables are included.

Eat Large Quantities of Vegetables
These will supply you with essential minerals and vitamins and provide fibre (roughage). Some people have become over-anxious about fibre, and have bran with everything. This is not a good idea, as it can irritate the bowel and hinder the absorption of some minerals. Eating vegetables is a better way to get fibre.

Eat Lots of Fresh Fruit
Although fruit contains quite a lot of sugar, it is in a different form from that in sweets (fructose rather than sucrose); it does not need insulin for its digestion and therefore is an ideal food to help slow down the pancreas.

Eat Some Fat
People tend to concentrate on low-fat diets (often dangerously low) and think this will take care of all cholesterol problems. However, there are other factors which are just as important – stress, and a diet low in raw vegetables and fruit can be just as damaging as moderate amounts of butter. Also remember that some foods actually lower cholesterol levels. They include onions, garlic, apples and olive oil. Olive oil is also wonderful for the immune system.

Suggested Diet

As soon as you get up: Small glass of unsweetened juice, or a piece of fruit.

Breakfast: More fruit juice and a cooked breakfast, such as grilled bacon, fish, eggs, baked beans, cold ham, cheese, or any protein dish, plus mushrooms or tomatoes.

Also one slice of wholemeal bread, two crispbreads, rice cakes etc. with butter or margarine. Alternatively, have whole oat porridge sweetened with a few sultanas; or muesli made from whole cereals, nuts, seeds (pumpkin, sunflower etc.); or plain yoghurt with fresh fruit and nuts (you could flavour this with spices such as cinnamon, ginger, crushed cardamom). Weak tea with milk if desired, or one cup of weak coffee.

Two hours after breakfast: A snack such as fruit, yoghurt, milk, cheese and biscuits.

Lunch: Any protein dish, hot or cold, such as meat, fish, cheese, eggs, chicken, sardines, tuna, pilchards etc., or any dish made from lentils, beans or nuts.

All to be eaten with *lots of salad or vegetables* and 1 slice of wholemeal bread or 2 crispbreads.

Two and a half to three hours after lunch: Weak tea, milk with crispbread, cheese, pâté or low-sugar jelly

Half an hour before dinner: Small glass of fruit juice.

Dinner: Same as lunch, plus fruit.

Supper: Crispbreads, butter, cheese, pâté, etc. Milk drink, weak tea, herb tea.

This might look like a lot of food, but remember there is no need to eat large quantities of each. Small and often is the rule.

General Points

- *Don't skip meals.*
- *Eat regularly.*
- *Avoid sugary foods and drinks.*
- *Avoid white flour.*
- *Cut down on caffeine, cigarettes and alcohol.*
- *Always have protein in your breakfast.*
- *Never eat a meal containing only starch (bread, cake, cereal).*

If you want to learn more about blood sugar problems, read *Low Blood Sugar (Hypoglycaemia)* by Martin L. Budd (Thorsons).

The Glycaemic Diet

The latest approach to eating to keep the blood glucose levels stable and therefore reduce cortisol levels – (see page 70) is the Glycaemic Diet: this is similar to the diet already discussed but places more of an accent on the ratio of protein to carbohydrate. The work of American Dr Elias Ilyia has proven that this eating plan reduces the stress on the body by balancing the level of insulin produced. It therefore reduces cortisol levels. Dr Ilyia suggests eating a ratio of one part protein to seven parts carbohydrate, although Dr Andrew Wright in his leaflet 'Glycaemic Eating' (available from The Complete Hormone Clinic – see Useful Addresses) suggests that it is more effective with a higher ratio of protein: one and half parts protein to two parts carbohydrate. His book on this diet stresses the importance of choosing 'good' – slowly absorbed – carbohydrates (such as whole grains) and gives recipes. This book is due to be published in 1999.

Although it might seem simplistic, eating to keep the blood sugar levels stable is the first step in lowering cortisol levels and therefore bringing DHEA levels into balance. By eating in a way which puts the pancreas under stress, you start the chain reaction which upsets the output of many other hormones. If you are anxious or have any stress-related symptoms *you cannot afford to ignore this*. You might say, 'but I have skipped breakfast, had a sandwich for lunch and a large evening meal for years' – exactly! You are paying the price for that now with anxiety, fatigue, mood swings and so on (see page 103). These are symptoms of hypoglycaemia. Try running your car without petrol or expecting an empty ink cartridge to print out your letters. This is exactly what you are doing to your body. It won't stand for this for ever and will complain with the symptoms mentioned. Hypoglycaemia also increases the risk of degenerative illnesses and maturity-onset diabetes.

18

Relaxation Training for Wayward Nerves

The importance of correct breathing, diet and exercise having been discussed, relaxation and using the mind to heal (creative visualization) are next.

What is Deep Relaxation?

Many people think they are relaxing when they curl up with a book or slump in a chair and watch television. These are enjoyable and restful things to do but do not constitute relaxation deep enough to promote a healing response – this has to be worked at. In order to relax deeply it is essential to:

1 *Be in a position where the spine is straight and supported.*
2 *Allow the joints and muscles to fall into natural positions.*
3 *Have the room at the right temperature.*
4 *Be free from distractions like telephones ringing or people talking.*
5 *Be able to let the mind wander.*
6 *Have an empty bladder.*
7 *Have neither an overfull nor an empty stomach.*

If you are tense it is quite possible that you do not relax even during sleep; your mind will be churning away and your body will be restless. (People who wake up stiff and sore can confirm how much muscular activity goes on in the night.) A deep relaxation session lasting about half an hour can be worth four hours of sleep.

Busy people should realize that incorporating a relaxation session into your day gives you more time, not less. Tension deprives joints, muscles and organs of normal blood flow and eventually affected areas will show their disapproval by becoming stiff, sore or possibly even diseased. Exercise and relaxation are the only ways you can guarantee that you are releasing the kinks and bottlenecks in the circulatory system and allow each cell to have its full ration of nutrients. If your headaches or your bowel symptoms are caused by tension consider *why* you are causing yourself this misery; why are you rushing around all the time? Why are you worrying constantly? Try to make the decision to stop.

Tension Release in Seconds

You can do this anywhere. Sit down with your back straight but not stiff, put your hands palm upwards in your lap and place your feet together flat on the floor. Droop your head a little, take one deep breath, and as you let it out let your shoulders drop and allow your thighs and knees to fall outwards. Imagine a beautiful, blue sparkling light about a foot above your head; let it ripple down through your body and out of the soles of your feet into the floor; it will take your tension with it. If you practise this regularly you will be surprised how effective it is. You may also notice it makes your feet tingle.

Creative Visualization

If you were taught biofeedback techniques by a therapist you would undoubtedly be delighted with the results: lower blood pressure, slower heartbeats and all the benefits of being more relaxed. With practice, in your own home, you can achieve the same results by using your own wonderful machine, your mind. By giving it positive images and loving, encouraging self-talk you can change useless worrying thoughts to helpful healing thoughts.

Here is an example of how the body follows the mind. You are sitting in the garden and you decide to do something active, play tennis or dig the vegetable garden for example. Just because you are *thinking* about being active, 'My tennis shoes are in the hall cupboard,' or 'Should I use the small fork or the new spade?' your brain has started to produce the chemicals you will need even before you have left your seat. This shows how you can use positive images to raise energy levels and improve performance. Conversely, negative images produce gloomy moods and tired muscles. To be able to use the mind effectively it needs to be quietened; you cannot relax if your mind is jumping hurdles.

Images Which Quieten the Mind

These images which follow are only suggestions; if they don't work for you, make up your own scene where there is cheerful noise and movement which becomes more and more tranquil. Here are some examples:

- *Imagine a tree filled with song birds. The birds fly away from the top branches, then the next branches, and so on until there is just one bird left. Concentrate on this bird until it flies off, then look at the branch it was sitting on and focus on just one lovely pale green leaf.*
- *Think of a fairground, full of laughter and music; it is closing down for the night. The people go home, the lights go out, and all becomes quiet.*
- *Imagine a playground of noisy, tumbling children. It's supper time; they gradually go home. Watch as the last child goes off with his mother; see how sleepy he looks.*

If you have trouble stilling your mind with images, try concentrating on the feeling in your nostrils as your breath enters and leaves, or simply by repeatedly counting to ten.

Thirty-Minute Relaxation Session

Some people are afraid to learn to relax because they use their tension as armour – it holds their fears and hurts (neuroses) inside, and keeps the frightening world out. But you cannot hold on to this tension and expect to be healthy. Neurosis is discussed in detail in my book *Coping with Anxiety and Depression* (see further reading).

It is a good plan to stimulate the circulation before you lie down, not only because it helps you to relax, but also because some people feel cold as tension eases. Keep a rug near you. If you become aware of your heartbeat or feel lightheaded as you relax don't be alarmed, just accept it; it is quite normal. Again, if you don't like the suggested imagery, find your own. The fountain could be replaced by a waterfall, your shower, water being poured from a jug, and the garden could, for example, be replaced by the shore, a meadow or your favourite room.

1   *Do a few stretching movements and have a good shake.*
2   *Lie on the floor or bed; to stretch the neck and to ensure the chin is not jutting forward, place a small firm pillow or a few paper-backed books under the head. Alternatively you can sit supported in a chair.*
3   *Breathe slowly and gently and imagine your body is sinking into the floor.*

Now begin your visualization. Imagine you are standing at a gate looking down on a lovely garden; inside the garden is wholeness, love and peace. You choose to open the gate and go inside. On the right there is a crystal clear fountain, the sun is shining through it and you can see all the colours of the spectrum. You feel the desire to be refreshed in the fountain and imagine as you stand underneath it that a beautiful flower about a foot above you opens and allows the water to wash through your head, taking with it any drug deposits, allergens or anything harmful to your brain, eyes, ears or sinuses. Then see it cleaning your throat and flowing down into your chest and abdomen, taking anything harmful to your body with it. Watch it as it goes down your legs and see a muddy stream leave the area under the arch of the foot. The muddy water goes deep into the ground. See your feet looking soft and clean.

Now watch the flower open again, and this time allow the water to wash through your mind, and release you from anything that has ever hurt you since before you were born: feelings of rejection, low self worth, grief, loneliness, unhappiness about your appearance, hurtful things people have said and done, guilt about how you have hurt others, frustrations, depression, anxiety, physical pain. Imagine it is all washing through you and leaving through your feet in a muddy stream; it completely disappears into the ground, leaving your feet looking soft and clean.

Now walk around the garden and notice if you feel lighter; you are wearing summer clothes and the grass is warm under your bare feet. You walk towards a yellow rose, and the colour surrounds your body; it fills you with tranquil feelings. Now you approach a white rose, you breathe in peace from its perfume. Your walk continues and you come to a thornless red rose bush. This rose fills you with love and forgiveness for yourself. See yourself as a little child; hug that child, stroke its hair, hold it and reassure it, tell it from now on you will do nothing to hurt it, give it another chance. See the child's face relax and smile and see the small figure, with loose limbs, clear skin and shining hair, skipping around the garden.

As you love and forgive yourself these feelings will extend to those around you. See the garden full of the people in your life and as you offer each one a rose let it be a symbol of love and forgiveness, their forgiveness of you and your forgiveness of them.

Now continue your walk in the garden, taking a gently sloping path down to the river. You pass the vegetable garden on the way and see cabbages and carrots growing – the soil looks fertile. When you reach the bottom you see a tree; there is a space in the branches where the sun is able to warm the ground. You lie down there and feel the rays of the sun travel over you. Feel a beautiful white light come over your feet; it makes them feel soft and warm. Imagine the light penetrating every cell of your body and let it travel to your calves, knees and thighs. Hold the light longer over the solar plexus area, and anywhere you experience pain or discomfort, and then let it travel up to the chest, shoulders, neck and head. Now imagine the whole body filled with healing white light; see it radiating several feet from your body. Say to yourself several times: 'Every day in every way I am getting better and better.'

Imagine you feel your energy level rising, and you stretch and slowly start to walk up the path to the rose garden, passing the vegetable garden again. Your step is very light. You pass the roses and the fountain and now you are at the gate. You come out of the garden. You can choose to go back there to be peaceful any time you wish.

Now wriggle your fingers and toes, then raise yourself onto your side before sitting up slowly.

If you practise visualization every day you will begin to feel things changing, you will become stronger and more in charge. You may be moving away from a lifetime of negative thoughts, so don't be too impatient – give it time. To many people the idea that they are valuable human beings worthy of love is very new, and visualizing themselves as children often brings tears. Welcome this if it happens: it is part of the healing you need. Also don't expect to forgive everyone in the first session; one woman said 'It took me nine weeks to give my ex-husband "a rose" but I felt so liberated when I managed it.'

You need not remember this guided imagery word for word, it is only a model for you to work from; you can make up any imagery you choose. The key factors to include are: being in a peaceful place; cleansing; looking at colours; loving and forgiving yourself and others; allowing a healing light to travel over you; and repeating a positive affirmation such as, 'every day etc.' or 'I love and approve of myself exactly as I am'; 'I am contented and healthy.' If you like the suggested imagery but have difficulty remembering it you could put it on tape. Some people find their own voice irritating on tape; if this is your experience ask a friend, particularly someone who cares for you, to do it for you.

Biofeedback

In biofeedback training electronic instruments feed back information to you about what is happening in your body. A lead is attached to the hand or head, or both. By means of a light getting brighter and dimmer, noise getting louder or softer, or by the position of a pointer on a screen, you can actually see what happens when you tighten and relax muscles or speed up and slow down your breathing. This enables you to become familiar with what your body feels like when your blood pressure is normal, when your pulse is steady and when your muscles are relaxed. The aim is to achieve this state without the machine. A course usually consists of half-hour sessions over an uninterrupted six to eight week period.

Biofeedback training is used in some NHS hospitals. You could ask your GP about it or you could buy a small biofeedback machine; they are often advertised in health magazines. Two leads are attached to your fingers and these measure the amount of tension; the machine emits a shrill sound if you are tense, and drops to a gentle clicking noise as you relax. You could also try Autogenic Training. Whilst it is better to have a teacher, if you really want to change, you can achieve very good results yourself.

Autogenic Training

This involves giving yourself positive commands when you are in a relaxed state. It differs from self-talk – which can be done anywhere at any time – and needs to be done in a disciplined manner. It can be used for relaxation, pain control, or for altering a negative and fixed mind-set (for example 'I cannot go out in case I can't find a lavatory in time').

Here is an example of a relaxation exercise; you can build in your own special commands at the end. Please note: *you will get much further with this if you do ten minutes abdominal breathing first, make sure you are warm, and that the telephone is disconnected.*

Repeat each command three times:
1   *My left arm is heavy and comfortable*
2   *My left leg is heavy and comfortable*
3   *My right arm is heavy and comfortable*
4   *My right leg is heavy and comfortable*
5   *My head is heavy and comfortable*

6 *My chest is heavy and comfortable*
7 *My abdomen is heavy and comfortable*
8 *My whole body is heavy and comfortable*

Repeat the entire sequence, this time giving the command.

My left arm is warm…
My digestion gets better every day – repeat eight times.
Every system in my body is balanced and healthy – repeat eight times.

Autogenic training is particularly useful for people who have difficulty conjuring mental images.

The Muscles of the Head and Neck

When we are tense we tighten up the sternomastoid muscle, which runs down the side of the neck, and this causes us to pull back our heads and jut the chin forward. This unnatural position causes a ripple of tension to go down the spine, through the pelvis, and even continue to the feet. This is why very tense people complain of 'jelly legs'. Imagine a column of dominoes set up; when the first one (the head) is tilted, the rest fall over. The importance of what you do with your head and shoulders cannot be overemphasized; after all, the head is such a heavy organ – about 14–21 lbs – that if it is not balanced, there is bound to be trouble.

How to Balance the Head

Sit on a chair with the spine straight, but not tensed. Look a few feet in front of you at the floor, (if your eyes are down you cannot shorten the muscles at the side of the neck), keeping your shoulders *down*, and raise your eyes enough to look comfortably around the room – this is the balanced position for your head. The chin is pointing downwards, not poking out in front. Whoever taught us to have our backs straight, heads up, shoulders back and chins up did us a great disservice; this is an unnatural position for the head and spine.

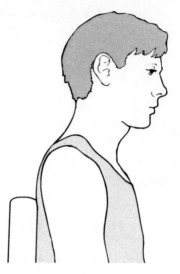

Fig. 3 Balanced position for the head

The Alexander Technique is one of the most successful methods of learning correct posture and how to move without tension. If you have a teacher near you it would be money well spent. Yoga is also very helpful.

Cutting Down the Blood Supply to the Head

When the neck and shoulder muscles are tight the effect is like putting a rubber band around the neck – the blood vessels are flattened and blood flow is restricted. Head problems such as migraine, sinusitis, tinnitus, irritability, feelings of unreality, lack of concentration, anxiety and depression can be the end result.

It is not surprising that there are important acupressure points for the digestion in the shoulders, as the position of the shoulders affects the digestion a great deal. The area between the shoulder blades on either side of the spine can be very tender in people who have the Irritable Bowel Syndrome.

Head, Neck and Shoulder Massage

You will need a partner for this and you will also need to *allow* him/her to help you; just sit there like a sack of potatoes and if you feel a little discomfort just try to bear it; it is an indication of how much you need those muscles moved.

Instructions for the helper

Areas of tension feel harder and resist the pressure of your fingers, so just work away in these areas and you will feel the muscles becoming less tight. Your fingers are bringing more blood to the area and allowing waste products to be taken away. Don't be too concerned about technique, if your thoughts are gentle towards your partner and you desire to help him/her you cannot do any harm; just follow these simple rules and let your fingers take over.

- Don't *massage over broken skin or varicose veins.*
- Don't *massage the front of the neck.*
- Don't *poke hard into muscles that feel hot and swollen.*
- Do *relax when you are massaging.*
- Do *allow your partner to do the same for you.*
- Do *remember to do shoulder exercises every day.*

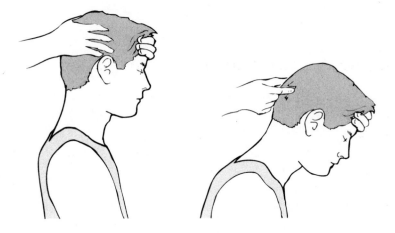

Fig. 4.1   Fig. 4.2

Be as relaxed as you can; let your breath out as you drop your shoulders; balance your partner's head, make sure his/her back is straight but slack, press her/his shoulders gently down.

1 *Support the forehead with one hand and move the muscles of the scalp just as if you were washing the hair with the other.*
2 *Continue to support the forehead and massage quite firmly at the base of the skull using the thumb and fingers to make small circular movements.*
3 *Now move onto the back of the neck using the thumb and index finger on either side of the neck bones; again using a circular movement.*
4 *Place your hands over the shoulders and use the thumb or heel of the hand to knead the muscles in a circular motion. Ask if there are any places needing extra attention.*
5 *Put one arm across the top of your partner's chest and encourage them to relax forward onto it. With the other hand continue massaging down the side of (but not on) the bones of the spine. Work in a similar fashion around the shoulder blade. Use the other arm and repeat for other side of spine.*
6 *Stand in front of your partner, pick up the wrist and shake the hand letting it flop (don't do this if there is pain in the joint);*

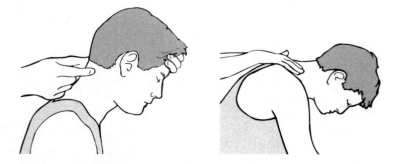

Fig. 4.3   Fig. 4.4

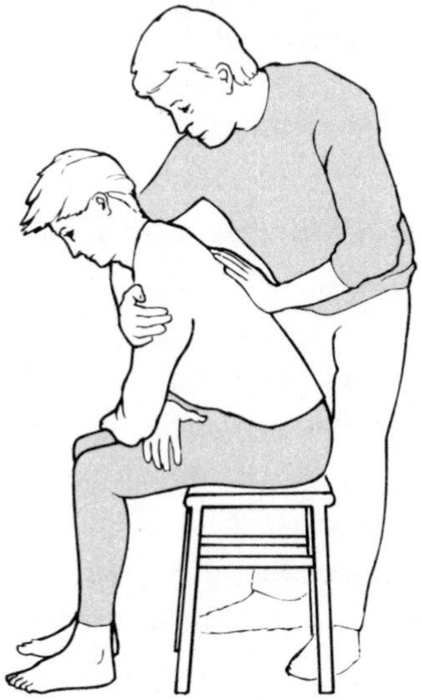

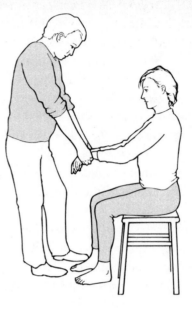

Fig. 4.5

Fig. 4.6

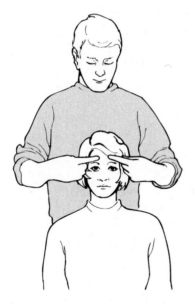

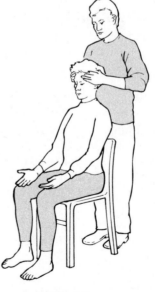

Fig. 4.7

Fig. 4.8

*and ask them to imagine a wet sweater on the washing line. You
will feel the arm become heavier when they think 'heavy'. Give
the hand a little shake then do the other hand and arm.*

7   *Stand behind your partner, support her/his head against your
chest and stroke the brow with both first fingers from the centre
outwards.*

8   *Finish off by stroking lightly and rapidly from the head down the
back and then down the arms and hands.*

Sometimes people are quite sleepy after a head and neck massage.
Your partner might need a short rest before helping you.

For the very tense person, it is a great help if they can have a
massage daily. The therapeutic value of massage is becoming more
recognized in this country. Aromatherapy – massaging with the
essential oils of plants – has been proved to have a beneficial effect
on the nervous system (see page 205).

The Solar Plexus

In physical terms the solar plexus is a collection of nerves just
below the diaphragm near the stomach and liver. We often react
emotionally in this area, and sometimes it is called the seat of the
emotions. Many of the expressions we use: 'gut feelings', 'I can feel
it in my gut', 'he dealt me a body blow', 'hitting below the belt', 'he
got me in the solar plexus', describe this. Tension in this area can
cause ulcers, constipation and period problems. The muscles of the
abdomen are also particularly important because they affect the
breathing.

Self-Massage for the Solar Plexus

When you are lying on the floor or bed:

1   *Breathe in slowly, and as you exhale press with the fingers of
both hands into the right groin.*

2   *Continue this, inching your way up the right side, across
and above the navel, pressing up into the ribs, and down the
left side.*

3 *Place hands flat, one just below the breast bone, the other with the lower edge just above the pubic bone, and vibrate them gently until your arms feel tired.*
4 *Hold your hands there, and imagine a golden ball of healing light filling your abdomen.*

19

The Bones –
Body Mechanics

The skeletal system provides a movable framework which gives support and protection to the soft tissues. The spine, which consists of thirty three irregular bones, serves as the main support of the trunk and neck, and gives protection to the spinal cord.

The Backbone

Although each joint in the backbone allows only slight movement, because there are so many of them the spine overall is flexible and allows the trunk to move freely – at least this is how it should be. Many people are afraid to move their spines and suffer back pain and sciatica as a result.

The backbone is connected to everything. The spinal nerves leave the spinal cord in pairs: nerves serving the neck and arms leave from the neck or cervical area; those serving the abdomen and rib-cage from the thoracic or chest area; those serving the lower back, hips and legs leave from the lumbar area; and the nerves serving the back of the legs leave from the sacral area. This should give you some idea of the area of the spine your symptoms may be coming from; a pain in the knee might have nothing to do with the knee but be coming from the spine, and a pain in the head or face can have its origins in the neck.

A Healthy Spine – A Healthy Body

Osteopaths and chiropractors believe that a straight, flexible spine means a healthy body and that slight displacements of vertebrae – called subluxations – interfere with the nerve supply and can cause organic disease. Sometimes local pain in the spine is not a feature, and malfunctions of the internal organs are the first sign. The symptoms caused by these displacements correspond to the vertebrae concerned; for example displacements of the atlas – the first bone of the spine – can impede the flow of blood in the vertebral arteries and cause migraine. The commonest causes of this displacement are repeated movements of the head to one side – to look at a badly-placed television set or notes at the side of a typewriter for example. Lying on the tummy in bed and keeping the head in one position is another cause.

Some chiropractors believe that displacements in the thoracic area can cause digestive and heart problems, and also allergies.

The Shoulder Bag Tilt

It is not usually anything dramatic which causes these displacements; using the body asymmetrically is the most common cause. Habitually using muscles on one side of the spine can pull the vertebrae sideways; for example always carrying the shopping or a child on one side, or reaching up to high shelves with the same hand, or taking your body weight mainly on one leg and one hip.

The Pelvic Tilt

The lower body takes the same punishment, and often the pelvis gets pushed up. This happens by bearing weight mainly on one side as you stand, or by continually letting the same leg take the impact of stepping down. The result of this habit can be back pain.

Because the pelvis is pushed up on one side it can appear that one leg is shorter than the other. You can check this by lying back in the bath, raising your feet and holding your ankles together. Look at your big toes, if they start and end at the same place then your pelvis is straight. If one toe looks shorter, then you could be pulling up on that side. This is very common and nothing to worry about unless you have back pain, in which case you could see an osteopath or chiropractor. To balance the pelvis and avoid future trouble, try standing on a box and swinging the short leg; or tying a belt or pair of tights around your ankle and instep, putting on a laced shoe or trainer, tying the other end to the leg of the bed, and then lying on the floor and shuffling back until you can feel some traction on that leg. Remember to weight-bear evenly if you have to stand and to step off the curb and down the first stair with the long leg.

Taking the Weight off the Spine

We often say we need to take the weight off our feet, when in fact it would be much better to relieve the spine of the crushing pressure of an unbalanced head. Ten minutes on the floor in the middle of the day, or whenever you are tired, can:

- *Take the pressure off the spine*
- *Allow the bones to fall into a natural position*
- *Improve the circulation.*

Stop! Just for ten minutes:

1   *Lie on your back with your knees bent and your feet flat on the floor.*
2   *Stretch your neck by placing a few paperback books or a firm pillow at the base of your skull.*
3   *Stay there for ten minutes then get up slowly.*

It would be ideal if you could imagine your spine becoming straight and flexible as you lie there, but if you cannot – and continue to work out your income tax or write mental shopping lists during the exercise – you will still benefit because of being in this position.

Daily Spinal Routine

Don't force yourself into any of these positions; just *breathe* yourself gradually into them. Once you begin to feel things happening you will get hooked on them and feel the difference if you don't do them; remember you will feel the effects throughout the whole body, not just in the spine.

Fig. 5. Stretching the spine – shiatsu style

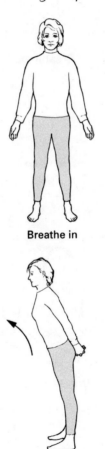

Breathe in

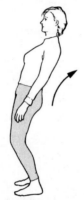

Breathe out

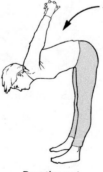

Breathe in

Breathe out

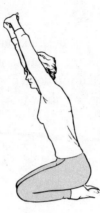
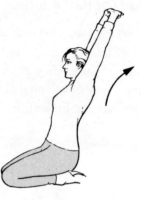

Breathe in

Breathe out

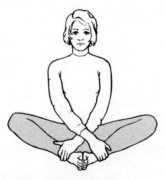
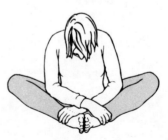

Breathe in

Breathe out

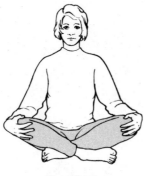

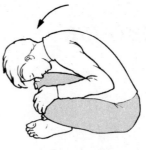

Breathe in   Breathe out

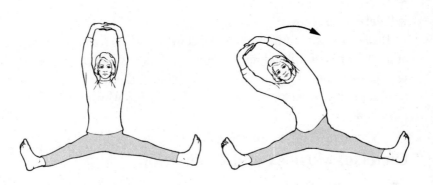

Breathe in   Breathe out

20

Exercise

It is often hard to convince people how important it is to exercise; they seem to think that because they feel low they should be as inactive as possible. If you do not have a fever, inflamed muscles, or any condition likely to be adversely affected by exercise, such as M.E. (check with your doctor if you are unsure), then *move*; you will delay your recovery if you don't.

Take care not to rush into frenetic activity if you have been sitting around for months. Build up the amount of exercise slowly. Some people are so out of touch with their bodies that they are very resistant to the idea of exercise. You will see below why it is so important:

Exercise, Muscles and Circulation

When you slow down your circulation by inactivity, organic function – for example the digestion – becomes sluggish; this causes constipation. Muscles are also affected, not only by lack of nourishment, but also by a build-up of crystals which are formed from the waste products of digestion. This is rather like soap powder collecting in the fibres of laundry that has not been adequately rinsed. The effect can be general muscle weakness and/or local congestion. Tension also locks these crystals into the muscles; a build-up in the shoulder area can be very painful and, in turn, cause you to move less. *If you do not move the muscles of the neck and shoulders, you restrict the blood supply to the head and give yourself endless problems.* You need to ask yourself, 'Am I causing my headaches, sinus problems, confusion?' The brain can become sluggish too, and when full circulation is restored symptoms of anxiety and depression can be dramatically relieved.

Exercise and the Lymphatic System

The lymphatic system is part of the body's defence system against disease. A body fluid called lymph, which relies on muscle contraction for its circulation, is carried through a complex network of small vessels which carry cellular refuse on the way. It is then passed into the bloodstream where it is processed. Unlike the circulatory system the lymphatic system has no pump; if you don't move then the lymph slows down. The results can be a collection of fluid in the tissues – particularly around the ankles if you have been sitting – a depressed immune system, and some cells in the body which rely on lymph for their nourishment becoming malnourished. Even if you have to stay in bed for some reason you can still help to circulate the lymph by gently squeezing each group of muscles in turn, and rotating the ankles and wrists. Massage can also be very helpful.

If you have been inactive for some time perhaps you could start with exercise while sitting down. As you do this routine, visualize anything that suggests improved circulation; slow streams becoming fast flowing sparkling rivers, pipes being unblocked – anything that comes to mind.

Exercises Sitting on a Chair

1   *Place your feet in front of you about a foot apart. Drop your shoulders and look at the floor a few feet in front of you; this stops you shortening the muscles at the side of the neck.*

2 Take one deep breath, lifting your shoulders as you do so; open your mouth as you let the breath out and drop your shoulders. Imagine you are as limp as a wet sweater.

3 Breathe normally, lift the shoulders towards the ears and let them drop towards the floor. Do this eight times if you can.

4 Keeping the arm limp, circle each shoulder in a front to back direction eight times, and then try doing them together.

5 To stretch the neck allow your head to fall to the right, bring it back to the centre, then allow it to drop to the left; four times each side. Don't raise your shoulder to meet your ear.

6 Stretch both arms to the ceiling and let them fall loosely towards the floor.

7 Stretch out the fingers, then draw eight circles both ways with the forefingers.

8 To exercise the legs draw the same circles with each big toe in turn.

9 For the buttocks and thighs tighten these muscles and feel yourself rise in your seat.

10 Finish by standing up and shaking all over like a wet dog.

Fear of being seen to shake in public can sometimes keep people indoors; regularly doing the wet dog exercise is very helpful. It takes a lot more energy to hold shaking in than to let it out. Have a good shake whenever you feel tense and particularly before any social event you are worried about. If you are in trouble when you are out find a lavatory where you can let your jaw go loose and allow yourself to shake from the head down.

Building Exercise into your Daily Life

See how many gentle stretching exercises you can incorporate in your daily routine: for example, walk upstairs on your toes to stretch the backs of your legs; reach up to shelves with both hands, hold the stretch then relax; do loose swinging movements, running on the spot, or the wet dog shake, when you are waiting for the kettle to boil; before getting into the bath hold the side and bend your knees a few times; rotate your ankles or massage your hands as you watch television.

Building these movements into your daily routine is useful if you do not feel up to swimming, walking or more strenuous exercise. Remember what happens to your circulation if you don't move. Perhaps the next stage could be walking briskly for thirty minutes daily and then progressing to aerobic exercise. It is easier and safer to have some supervision. Join a class or take the advice of the fitness coach at a leisure centre. The exercises might feel like a terrible chore at first but just keep going; when you feel the benefits you will be more enthusiastic. See the reference list for medical research on exercise and health.

21

The Importance of Daylight

There has been a lot of interest in the last decade in the effect of light on human health. Biologists have discovered that not only is it vital for our well-being, but also that individual requirements for light vary as much as individual needs for vitamins. As humans have become more civilized they have spent less time outdoors; many people travel to work by car to badly-lighted buildings and then return home by car to spend an evening indoors watching television. We do not wilt visibly like plants in a dark corner, but there is no doubt that the shorter days of the autumn and winter do adversely affect some people. They experience lethargy, loss of interest in sex, and depression; as daylight increases in the spring these feelings disappear and normal energy levels return. While many people can say they feel a little let down in the winter, there are some people who are so seriously affected by light reduction that they have a condition known as Seasonal Affective Disorder (SAD). Sufferers become extremely depressed, have joint pains and digestive problems, crave sweet foods and lack concentration sometimes to the extent that they cannot continue their studies or work. They have great difficulty getting out of bed in the mornings and are exhausted all day.

Fortunately it has been found that being exposed to light which replicates daylight for several hours a day cures this condition. When this light, or real daylight, enters the eye it stimulates the pineal gland and inhibits the production of a substance called melatonin. Normally melatonin is only produced at night in the dark; this is what makes us sleepy.

Daylight is necessary for normal brain functioning and for the regulation of the sleep-wake cycle, so you can see that staying indoors when you are depressed or ill in any way can only compound your problems. Even if you are severely agoraphobic you could sit at an open window without any glasses; do this for a minimum of twenty minutes daily in the brightest part of the day.

Sunlight

While it is foolish to risk skin cancer or ageing the skin prematurely by baking in the sun for hours, it is equally foolish to be always covered in sun block and never allow the sun to reach the skin. Frequent exposure for short periods has many beneficial effects, including the production of Vitamin D. We look healthier after a little sun and this increases feelings of well-being, and sunlight also kills bacteria and fungus.

Fresh Air

Unless they actually have chest problems, it is often difficult to convince people of the benefits of good breathing habits, and even harder to impress upon them the dangers of continually filling the lungs with stale air. Air that is contaminated by smoke and fumes is recognized as being harmful; but there can be other causes of stale air that are not so well known.

Positive Ions

Electrically polluted air can be the cause not only of respiratory problems but also of headaches, irritability, digestive problems and depression. Particles in the air around us – called ions – are electrically charged, positive and negative. We breathe in these particles and absorb them through the skin. If the air is overloaded with positively charged particles it can have a powerful effect on the nervous system. The brain overproduces a chemical called serotonin, and this can produce nasal congestion, lethargy, feeling sticky (not the same feelings as being too hot) and swollen. The oppressive feeling before an electrical storm best describes this, a restless feeling – being 'under the weather'. We can also experience this in cities where stale air is trapped between tall buildings or in workplaces where the air is filled with positive ions from VDUs (see Useful Addresses). At home this effect can be felt if we sit in badly ventilated rooms surrounded by plastic and electrical equipment, wearing clothes made from synthetic fibres.

Geological location and climate are also factors which affect the air. Warm winds – like the Mistral in the Mediterranean and the Santa Anna in California – are loaded with positive ions, and are dreaded by many people because they make them feel enervated and depressed.

Negative Ions

Negative ions have a tonic effect on the nervous system and reduce histamine levels in the blood. As any allergy sufferer knows, histamine is strongly associated with unpleasant feelings. The benefits of negative ionization are becoming widely known, not only for cleaning the air, killing bacteria and viruses, but also as a treatment for asthma, bronchitis, migraine, burns, scalds and wounds. Sufferers from the Irritable Bowel Syndrome could also benefit from negatively charged air. An interesting book called *The Ion Effect* (Fred Soyka, Bantam, 1978) describes the effect of positive ions on the bowel.

Weather-Sensitive People

After a thunderstorm the air is negatively charged; it smells fresh and we experience 'the calm after the storm', our energy returns and our mood improves. The air by the sea, by waterfalls and flowing water, even by the shower, is also negatively charged and can produce a feeling of well-being. Some people are more affected by this than others, in the same way that some people are irritable and restless when the moon is full and others do not notice it. At full moon the positively charged layer of the ionosphere – the layer of air and particles which absorbs harmful radiation from the sun – is pushed nearer the earth, thus increasing the number of positive ions in the air we breathe.

Avoid Being Bombarded with Positive Ions

Keep your home well ventilated and avoid nylon sheets, carpets and clothes if possible. At work, take frequent breaks from VDU screens, fit a screen protector and buy an ionizer (a small machine that negatively charges the air). Ionizers are available in most large stores, but you may have to look in a health magazine for an address for a VDU screen protector. If you drive a lot you could fit a small ionizer in the car. This greatly reduces the effects of pollution and car sickness. Many drivers have reported that they feel less tired at the end of the day.

Can I Overdo Negative Ions?

No, there is no maximum dosage, you can breathe in as many as you like. Some people have ionizers in every room. If you have one in your sitting room don't forget to put it by your bed at night; they do help you to have a restful night.

22

The Health of the Electrical Field

We are Electrical Beings

A biophysicist called Dr Walter Stark believes that the body absorbs ions at acupressure points. This brings us to an area of health that is rarely discussed; we talk about the health of the circulatory system, the state of the nervous system and so on, but what about the health of our electromagnetic fields?

Our hearts, brains, muscles and nerves all run on a delicate form of electricity, so it follows that, while we do not need to be plugged into a socket in the wall to operate, we are still electrical beings and are surrounded by an electromagnetic field. In the 1930s a Russian named Kirlian experimented with photography which clearly showed this field. One of the first people to study what he called the L-fields or the fields of life, and how they affect health, was Harold Saxon Burr of Yale University Medical School. Dr Robert O. Becker, author of *The Body Electric*, and a leading modern researcher on electromagnetic pollution, believes that artificial electromagnetic fields from power lines and electrical appliances can cause depression, a depressed immune system and other health problems. Becker's research and the work of others suggests that disturbances in the electrical field develop before illness in the physical body. This could be the medicine of the future – the prevention and treatment of illness through correcting faults in the electromagnetic field. This knowledge is not new, and similarities can be found in ancient forms of healing. Because of the work of American nurse Dolores Kreiger, a technique which clears and energizes the electromagnetic field is taught in some nursing schools; it is known as Therapeutic Touch. She describes this in her book *Therapeutic Touch, How To Use Your Hands to Help or Heal*, published by Prentice-Hall.

Can I Feel my Own Electrical Field?

Only 1 per cent of people can't – try it. You might have to try on a few occasions before you can be sure, but the more you practise, the more sensitive your hands will become. The movement used to build up the field between the hands is like that of playing a concertina slowly:

1 *Sit in an upright chair with your back straight but not tense, drop your shoulders and breathe slowly from the abdomen. If you can continue to do this while you are following the rest of the exercise it would be better, but if you cannot fit it in with the rest just do a few slow breaths before you start.*

2 *Stretch your fingers out wide and become aware of the palms of your hands.*

3 *Rub your hands together briskly for about fifteen seconds.*

4 *Hold your hands about eight inches apart then gradually bring them towards each other until they are about one inch apart; do not let them touch.*

5 *Separate the hands again, this time to about six inches apart and then bring them towards each other, again without touching.*

6 *Separate them once more, and this time bring them together again and bounce them together, remembering to keep the hands relaxed. You will feel a resistance or a feeling of pressure between your hands. Some people say they feel as if there is foam rubber*

between their hands, others describe feelings of heat, tingling, throbbing or pulling.

Using Your Hands to Clear Positive Ions from Your Field

Now that your hands are energized you can use them to clear congestion, increase relaxation, and ease discomfort.

1   *Rub your feet and massage under the arch for about a minute. If your feet are very tense take a little longer over this, then place them flat on the floor if sitting.*
2   *Sit relaxed or lie on the floor or bed; slow down your breathing.*
3   *Close your eyes and imagine yourself totally well and peaceful. If you cannot conjure up this image, give yourself the command:*

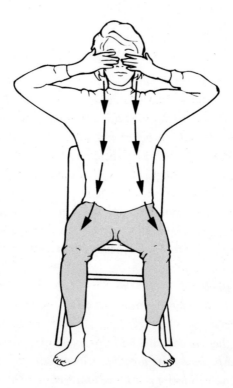

Fig. 6

'I am totally well and peaceful,' and imagine a pure white light is entering your head, filling your body and coming from your fingers and palms. Reach up beyond your head and stroke about three to four inches above your body just as though you were touching it; move down over your face, neck, chest and abdomen and then sweep the hands to either side of the body; this is important because you need to take the congestion clear of your body. You will feel prickling or heat in your hands as you pick up congestion. You can just flick this off as though you are shaking water from your hands.

4   Continue stroking for about ten minutes or until your arms feel tired.

5   Now, still imagining you are filled with white light and seeing it coming from your hands, hold them over your abdomen and imagine your digestive tract and all your internal organs becoming healthy and vitalized.

Increasing Energy in Selected Areas

In this part of the exercise you are sending energy to an area of discomfort. You may feel heat or cold and possibly rumblings in your gut. Don't be surprised if it makes loud noises. This is just a sign that you are relaxing. As you practise this you will get a feeling of being 'finished'. That is the only way to describe the sensation of an area having taken enough energy. You might also notice your nose feeling less congested or your sinuses making popping noises when you are working around your head. You can transfer energy in the same way to any aching muscles or joints that you can reach. Clearing congestion from the field also helps to cool a fever, ease itching and reduce swelling.

Many people get very enthusiastic about Therapeutic Touch and are keen to use it to help others. This is certainly to be encouraged but not before you are well and have learned more about it. Unfortunately most of the reading on this subject is American and some of the books are difficult to get in the UK. Dolores Kreiger's *Therapeutic Touch, How to Use Your Hands to Help or Heal* is probably the most readily available.

23

Vitamins and Minerals

It is always best to be guided by a doctor or nutritionist about the supplements you need, but if this is not possible, here is some information on the supplements most commonly used. A hundred years ago this information would not have been necessary, but alas, the days when a good diet was the only precaution necessary against nutritional deficiencies have gone. The awful things that we do to food and to ourselves – polluted food, processed food, fad diets, hindrance of absorption by alcohol consumption, medical drugs and street drugs, as well as heavy consumption of tea and coffee all cause nutritional deficiencies. When you see how many of the vitamins and minerals depend on each other for their full use, you will see that it is essential to have a varied diet and a clean bowel in good working order.

Supplements should be regarded as a medicine; take them for a time (unless otherwise instructed by your physician) until health is restored; after that the situation should be reviewed.

The B Vitamins

If the B vitamin status of the nation was better fewer prescriptions for tranquillizers would be issued and there would be fewer worried, tired, sad people around. But before you rush out for a bottle of B complex there are a few things to learn that might be helpful.

Some of the Problems with the Bs

If you can tolerate a good quality vitamin B complex then all is well; take it until you feel better (it may take as long as three months before some of your deficiencies are balanced), then take it intermittently when you feel you need it – once your bowel is clean and your diet is sound you may not need it at all.

Unfortunately many people who have allergies, or digestive problems, cannot tolerate B complex, even if they use the purest hypoallergenic products. They complain of headaches, heavy muscles, bloating and hyperactivity, and some suffer severe insomnia. When you change the nutritional state of the body some symptoms must be expected.

Some people find they can continue if they take a very small portion of the tablet and then increase slowly, others put up with the discomfort and after about three weeks things improve. With others the answer seems to be taking each B vitamin separately and finding out which one causes the trouble. This latter method makes quite a lot of sense in other ways, because many of the Bs have specific effects which can be used very successfully (for example, B_4 can be a powerful tranquillizer). Because all the books warn against taking separate B vitamins in isolation – because many of them need each other to function and also because of the risk of depleting the store of the others if only selected ones are taken – perhaps one answer would be to have a good dietary intake, keep trying with the B complex and use specific ones in addition. For example if you had chilblains you could take extra niacin or if you were dealing with *Candida* you could take extra biotin. When they are all taken together the stimulating ones can make an anxious person feel even worse and so some of the valuable therapeutic effects are lost.

Dr Douglas Hunt in his book *No More Fears – A New Nutritional Programme to Free You from Phobias and Irrational Fears* (Thorsons), gives combinations of vitamins and minerals for facing difficult situations such as exams or going out if you are agoraphobic. It is not a good idea randomly to take a few of these and a few of those. If you want effects other than the general improvement in nutrition which results from taking a multimineral and a multivitamin product, you will either have to have professional help or really do your homework.

You will see below some of the reasons for the body running low on essential nutrients. In addition to those mentioned, remember that the body's needs for all nutrients increases enormously during times of emotional stress such as bereavement, overwork or relationship difficulties, and also during times of physical stress such as infections, injuries, surgery and pregnancy.

Vitamin B₁ (Thiamine)

Functions:	Normal growth; digestion; healthy nerves; healthy heart
Sources:	Widely available in the diet; wholegrains, meat, fish, pulses, nuts, eggs, most vegetables
Causes of Deficiency:	Poor diet (too much pure carbohydrate such as alcohol), dirty colon, colon disorders such as the Irritable Bowel Syndrome
Deficiency Signs and Symptoms:	Fatigue, loss of appetite, nervous tension (build up of lactic acid in the brain) phobias, confusion, constipation, pins and needles, sensitivity to noise, impairment of sense of touch, retention of fluid. *Severe deficiency*: beriberi – disorder affecting muscles and brain; tingling or burning in legs, tender calf muscles, double vision, nystagmus (involuntary movements of eyeballs), paralysis of muscles around eyes.

Vitamin B$_2$ (Riboflavin)

Functions:	Helps the body use carbohydrates and protein; helps in alcohol and yeast sensitivity
Sources:	Wholegrains, pulses, liver, milk, eggs, leafy greens, brewer's yeast
Causes of Deficiency:	Dirty colon, colon disorders, major tranquillizers, probably minor tranquillizers and sleeping pills (valium group), tricyclic antidepressants, alcoholism, slimming. Not a huge amount available in the diet, and so is quite a common deficiency (the most common one in the United States). Recovery from deficiency is slow.
Deficiency Signs and Symptoms:	Dizziness, shaking, pre-menstrual tension (PMT), sore eyes, gritty eyes, twitching of eyelids. *Severe deficiency*: corneal damage, cataract, anaemia, weak muscles.

Vitamin B$_3$ (Niacin)

Functions:	Health of all cells, essential for digestion (works with enzymes); needed for healthy skin; nerves and sex hormones; cleans out toxins; helps circulation; helpful in allergies and sugar and alcohol cravings
Sources:	Wholegrains, lean meat, liver, poultry, fish, nuts, pulses
Causes of Deficiency:	Dirty colon, disorders of liver and colon, alcoholism, stress, lack of B$_6$
Deficiency Signs and Symptoms:	Dry lips, fissured tongue, wind, Irritable Bowel Syndrome, anxiety, depression, high blood cholesterol, hardening of the arteries, skin sensitive to sunlight or friction. *Severe deficiency*: pellagra (rough skin)

Note: This is a very useful supplement for people who are always cold, for chilblains, and as a tranquillizer. There is often a harmless skin prickling or flush after taking it. This does not last long and is good for the circulation. The synthetic vitamin B_3 (nicotinamide) does not have this effect; it is also less sedating, and because of this might be more helpful if you are depressed.

Vitamin B_4 (Choline)

Functions:	Health of nerves is the main effect; one of the most important messengers in the brain; also necessary for vitamin B_1 to work; helps in the breakdown of fat
Sources:	Egg yolk, liver, brewer's yeast, wholegrains, lethicin (which has no tranquillizing effect because it contains phosphorus which is a stimulant)
Causes of Deficiency:	Poor diet
Deficiency Signs and Symptoms:	Dizziness, visual problems, nervousness.

Vitamin B_5 (Pantothenic Acid)

Functions:	Growth; enzyme production; makes cortisone and sex hormones; needed for the absorption of other B vitamins; helps the body excrete lactic acid; helps stabilize blood sugar levels
Sources:	Widely available in the diet; wholegrains, vegetables, animal foods, brewer's yeast, royal jelly
Causes of Deficiency:	Lack of other B vitamins, dirty colon, colon disorders

Deficiency Signs and Symptoms:	Low blood sugar, headaches, chest infections, lowered antibody production, sore joints, poor muscle co-ordination, premature greying of the hair, gastric ulcers, tingling and numbness in limbs, cramp

Folic Acid

Functions:	Essential for normal metabolism; helps make red blood cells; keeps hormone levels stable; helps PMT and tiredness
Sources:	Green leafy vegetables, liver, kidney; made in the bowel
Causes of Deficiency:	Dirty colon, old age, pregnancy, antibiotics, poor diet
Deficiency Signs and Symptoms:	Anaemia, psoriasis, sore tongue, digestive problems *Severe deficiency*: some forms of psychosis.

Vitamin B₆ (Pyridoxine)

Functions:	Absorption of protein; proper growth; works with niacin and essential fatty acids (EFAs); immune system; skin; digestion and hormone production
Sources:	Wholegrains, liver, fish, chicken, potatoes, bananas, avocados; made in small amounts in a healthy gut
Causes of Deficiency:	Dirty colon, colon disorders, stress, dieting, alcoholism
Deficiency Signs and Symptoms:	Dizziness, hot, crawling or tingling sensations in the skin, deficiency of antibodies, tendency to allergies, tendency to phlebitis, cracks at the angle of the mouth, swollen taste buds, greasy redness at the sides of the nose, depression, sore breasts, retention of fluid, irritability, anaemia.

Caution: some people have taken B$_6$ in doses over 500 mg daily over a prolonged period for PMT. Resulting damage to the nervous system can cause: unsteadiness, numbness and clumsy movements of the hands.

Vitamin B$_{12}$ (Cyanocobalamin)

Functions:	Health of red blood cells and the functioning of all cells and bone marrow; growth; essential for health of nervous system; necessary for the absorption of folic acid
Sources:	Animal foods, eggs
Causes of Deficiency:	Lack of substance in the stomach called the intrinsic factor, bowel disorders, strict diet
Deficiency Signs and Symptoms:	Sore mouth and tongue, dry scaly skin, bumpy rash on upper arm, tingling of hands and feet, depression, poor memory. *Severe deficiency:* pernicious anaemia – exhaustion, brain and spinal cord affected.

Biotin (formerly called vitamin H)

Functions:	Works with enzymes; essential for the utilization of EFA's and carbohydrates; helps clean up after proteins have been used; suppresses the growth of the invasive form of *Candida* in the bowel
Sources:	Liver, nuts, beans, egg yolks, cauliflower; made in healthy gut by bacteria
Causes of Deficiency:	Dirty colon, disorders of the colon, stress, prolonged consumption of raw eggs (protein called avidin in eggwhite prevents absorption), antibiotics, sulphonamide drugs, genetic defect causing malabsorption

Deficiency Signs and Symptoms:	Tiredness, sore lips and tongue, digestive problems, difficulty swallowing, scaly dermatitis, depression, hair loss.

Other Vitamins

Vitamin C (Ascorbic acid)

Functions:	Growth; healing; detoxification; dealing with free radicals;* immune system; wound healing
Sources:	Most fruit and vegetables
Causes of Deficiency:	Poor diet, smoking, stress, injury, pollution, contraceptive pill
Deficiency Signs and Symptoms:	Lack of energy, aches and pains, swollen gums, spontaneous bruising, slow healing of wounds, repeated infections, poor colour, anaemia. *Severe deficiency*: Scurvy – swollen bleeding gums, internal bleeding, weak bones.

Note: can be used in quite large doses for specific effects, such as detoxifying, boosting the immune system, helping constipation, as a stimulant, and to neutralize food intolerance reactions. It is also a good hangover cure. If it is taken regularly in large doses, a good multimineral supplement should be taken as well, as vitamin C washes minerals out.

Free Radicals: these are delinquent oxygen molecules found in blood and tissue which are strongly suspected of causing degeneration and cancer. Some are released as part of the immune defence of the body, and some come from sources outside the body, such as tobacco smoke, organic solvents, food additives, pesticides, heavy metals, radiation.

When fats combine with oxygen they become rancid and cannot be fully digested, and this releases more free radicals. When the body fights bacteria it makes its own free radicals and it also makes a substance, derived from what we eat, to neutralize them. This is why it is so important to eat the substances that provide the raw material for this job. They include: vitamin C, vitamin E, beta-carotene (the vegetable form of vitamin A), the minerals selenium and zinc, and the amino acids L-cysteine and L-methionine. It is also important to keep intake of animal fats low.

Vitamin D

Functions:	Helps in the absorption of calcium; essential for bones and teeth
Sources:	Oily fish, liver, dairy products, egg yolk; made by the action of the sun on the skin
Causes of Deficiency:	Poor diet, lack of sunlight
Deficiency Signs and Symptoms:	Soft bones (if severe in children development of bow legs), backache, aching limbs, muscle weakness, weak bones, fractures.

Vitamin E

Functions:	Vital for the health of cells; slows down ageing; fights free radicals
Sources:	Vegetable oils, wheatgerm, wholemeal cereal, green leafy vegetables
Causes of Deficiency:	Absorption problems, poor diet
Deficiency Signs and Symptoms:	Fatigue, poor skin. *Severe deficiency*: shortness of breath, palpitations, anaemia.

Caution: some people have had withdrawal symptoms – cut down gradually.

Vitamin K

Functions:	Necessary for blood to clot (often called anti-haemorrhagic vitamin); used after surgery and during labour to prevent blood loss
Sources:	Green leafy vegetables, fruits, seeds, root, cow's milk, yogurt, alfalfa;* also made in the bowel
Causes of Deficiency:	Bowel troubles, especially chronic diarrhoea
Deficiency Signs and Symptoms:	Tendency to bleed. *Severe deficiency:* bleeding from the intestine or urinary tract.

*Alfalfa seeds are often sprouted and eaten in salads. An Oxford therapist has had considerable success for many years using alfalfa tablets or capsules for the Irritable Bowel Syndrome.

Minerals

Calcium

Calcium controls the effects of all other major minerals (potassium, magnesium, sodium) and the amino acids; the health of the cell is very dependent on it. It also carries messages around the inside of the cell and activates nerve signals. It is vital for our mental health and generally has a calming effect. A multimineral is often prescribed with calcium. If you are taking calcium for anxiety it is better not to take magnesium in doses above 200mg daily, as it can act as a stimulant. Also watch this if you have diarrhoea.

Functions:	Health of all cells, bones and teeth; nerves; blood clotting
Sources:	Dairy produce, green leafy vegetables, beans, nuts, sardines, drinking water in some areas, raisins, bancha tea*
Causes of Deficiency:	Poor diet, pregnancy, breast feeding, lack of vitamin D

| Deficiency Signs and Symptoms: | Soft bones, joint pains, panic attacks, hyperactivity, muscle spasm. |

* Bancha tea is a healthy drink with a pleasant smokey flavour. Many tea drinkers find after they have become accustomed to bancha a cup of their old brew tastes bitter and unpleasant. It is an alkaline drink and can be made in the familiar way or simmered in a pan. The leaves can be re-used. Use 1–2 tablespoonful in a pan with two pints of water. Strain and serve, preferably without milk.

Magnesium

Functions:	Bones, teeth and transmission of nerve impulses; regulation of body temperature; contraction of muscles; conversion of blood to energy
Sources:	Wholegrains, nuts, some drinking waters, sea foods, soya
Causes of Deficiency:	Constant diarrhoea or vomiting, alcoholism, dirty colon, some water tablets (diuretics), contraceptive pill
Deficiency Signs and Symptoms:	Muscle spasm, ringing in ears, anxiety, depression, palpitations, shaking. *Severe deficiency:* claw-like spasm of hands and feet; may allow calcium to be deposited in the kidney causing kidney stones; may cause predisposition to heart disease.

Potassium

Functions:	Works with sodium to control fluid balance of the body
Sources:	Green leafy vegetables, oranges, apples, potatoes, bananas, lean meat
Causes of Deficiency:	Water tablets, diarrhoea or vomiting, long term steroids, abusing laxatives, large quantities of tea or coffee

| *Deficiency Signs and Symptoms:* | Muscle weakness, dizziness, confusion, constipation, impairment of nerve function. |

Sodium

Functions:	Water balance; muscle contraction and nerve impulses; keeps heart rhythm steady
Sources:	Widely available in the diet
Causes of Deficiency:	Prolonged diarrhoea or vomiting, heat stroke, burns, heavy physical work causing profuse sweating
Deficiency Signs and Symptoms:	Lethargy, dizziness, cramps, palpitations.

Note: too much salt causes increased risk of heart disease and high blood pressure; fluid retention.

Iron

Functions:	Forms red blood cells and is vital part of the pigment haemoglobin which carries oxygen around the body; converts blood sugar to energy
Sources:	Liver, meat, chicken, eggs, fish, green leafy vegetables, pulses, wholegrains, dried fruit
Causes of Deficiency:	Heavy periods, pregnancy, poor diet, vegetarian diets (the vegetable sources of iron are harder to absorb than the animal sources), gastric ulcers
Deficiency Signs and Symptoms:	Anaemia, pallor, fatigue, shortness of breath, encourages growth of *Candida*, irritability, lowered resistance to infection.

Zinc

Functions:	Vital in enzyme activity; needed for health of all cells and for healing of wounds and burns
Sources:	Meat, nuts, seeds, pulses, wholegrains, seafoods
Causes of Deficiency:	Poor diet, dieting, adolescence, old age, bowel disorders, alcoholism; tranquillizers and sleeping pills are known to block the absorption of zinc (and it is likely that other minerals and vitamins are lost as well); profuse sweating
Deficiency Signs and Symptoms:	Acne, inflamed eyes, sore mouth and tongue, slow healing of wounds, white spots on nails, inflammation around nails, anxiety, depression, loss of appetite, anorexia nervosa, hair loss.

Other Nutrients

Essential Fatty Acids *(Polyunsaturates – Vitamin F)*

Functions:	Essential for the health of the whole body; not made by the body and must be taken in the diet
Sources:	Vegetable oils, fish oils, evening primrose oil*
Causes of Deficiency:	Processing of ingested oil (such as heating), poor diet, deficiency of nutrients necessary for absorption (B_6, zinc, vitamin C, vitamin B_3), drugs, alcohol, ageing
Deficiency Signs and Symptoms:	Fatigue, irritability, general ill health, joint pain, skin problems, hair loss, premature ageing

* Evening Primrose Oil: the seeds of this plant (used by the American Indians for healing) produces a pure oil rich in EFAs. It is being used more and more for a variety of problems and is now available on prescription for eczema. Some of its benefits are:

- *Lowers cholesterol*
- *Keeps blood vessels healthy*
- *Helps insulin to work*
- *Prevents inflammation and controls arthritis*
- *Relieves PMT*
- *Lowers blood pressure*
- *Helps in loss of excess weight*
- *Used in the treatment of multiple sclerosis, alcoholism, allergies, hyperactivity, anxiety and depression, skin problems*
- *Retards ageing*
- *Thought to prevent cancer.*

Here is an extract from Dr Caroline Shreeve's book *The Premenstrual Syndrome* (Thorsons) about how evening primrose oil helps PMT and other conditions. Note that deficiency of essential fatty acids is not rare:

The prolactin level itself is normal; and so, often, are the measured levels of oestrogen and progesterone. But because the body is *lacking in EFAs* [my emphasis] it is hypersensitive to the normal level of prolactin which is present. Instead of having too much prolactin, the affected women have too few EFAs, but with respect to the premenstrual symptoms this amounts to the same thing. B_6 increases the efficiency with which the body tissues make use of the EFAs. So, a person taking a supplement of pyridoxine is able to utilize the supply of EFAs that is available to her, to the best advantage.

Efavite is a product made to take with evening primrose oil; it contains all the necessary nutrients to convert the raw material of the oil into a very valuable healing substance. (For more information read *Evening Primrose Oil* by Judy Graham (Thorsons).)

24

Some Reasons for not Getting Better

Some people are not really prepared to change habits, yet they expect results. If you don't follow the rules (good nutrition, exercise, etc.); if you drink alcohol excessively; if you smoke; and if you refuse to control tension, then you can forget it, you will not recover. But there are other traps you can fall into, some of which follow.

Rushing Around Like a Paper Kite

Many people, because they feel well for the first time for years after making some basic changes, simply do too much; they get so absorbed in working again they forego relaxation and fresh air; they start to neglect their diet and then wonder why they feel ill again. They cry, 'I'm anxious and aching all over and my gut is playing up again.' Of course it is. If the nervous system is strained it complains, and remember if you want to stay well you may never be able to abuse your nervous system the way you used to. The lesson you have had should have been painful enough for you never to risk over-stimulated nerves again.

Mistaking Hyperactivity for Being Well

Some hyperactive people mistakenly think they are well, because in spite of getting very little sleep they have boundless energy. Activity can only be said to be healthy when your muscles respond with fatigue, and recover with rest. In the short-term the hyperactive person does not feel the need for rest; but the body will eventually respond with exhaustion and frayed nerves.

Lack of Exercise

Are you holding yourself back, tense, because you are too afraid to really move? Your gut problems, anxiety, depression and aching muscles will not go until you take this possibility seriously. Build up an exercise programme gradually until you are doing really tiring exercises at least three times weekly. If you have any doubts about how much you should do consult your doctor.

Hanging onto Your Anxiety/Depression

The responsibility for your emotional state is yours. Outside factors may make life very hard for you, but what actually goes on in your body is determined by *you*; if you respond to life with tension, this causes anxiety which in turn causes depression. This is not being done to you, you are doing it and what is more, it is a habit that needs a great deal of determination to break. It is true that when you feel ill you need understanding and support, but subsequently it is up to you to take responsibility and train yourself to live without tension.

Refusal to Look at the Psychological Side

Being physically low often acts as a catalyst; all the stored rubbish from the unconscious is unearthed because the person is too weak to hold it in. This does not happen to everyone, because some people are able to express their emotions as they experience them. While many people recover as soon as the physical cause of their discomfort is eased, there are others who don't. Often these are people who stubbornly refuse to acknowledge that there could be psychological problems too. Hanging on to guilt, anger, frustration and failure to forgive will keep you firmly on the tension–anxiety anxiety-depression trail.

Illness Used to Manipulate Relationships

Some people are afraid (albeit subconsciously) of losing love or power if they become well. For example a person may get a great deal more attention, be safe from anger and feel secure in the knowledge that their partner will not leave them, if they are sick. Sometimes a person will also stay sick to punish a partner for old misdeeds.

25

Quick References: Symptoms and Action

Diarrhoea

Acute:

1 *Rest.*
2 *Take fluids only; no milk or citrus, minimal tea or coffee.*
3 *Consult doctor if it persists.*

Chronic:

1 *Consult doctor. If this is not helpful investigate possible causes (food allergy, Candida, fear, drugs).*
2 *Cut down on fluids, avoid milk and citrus drinks.*
3 *Take a bulking agent (linseed, Isogel).*
4 *Eat a clean, varied diet.*
5 *Look after your nerves: slow down, take up relaxation exercises, self-talk, counselling, recreation, laughter.*
6 *Look after your general health: exercise, daylight and fresh air.*
7 *Practise delaying going to the lavatory.*

Constipation

1 *Increase fluids; take as little milk as possible, cut down on tea and coffee.*
2 *Eat lots of fruit and vegetables.*
3 *Take linseed or bulking agent with lots of water.*
4 *Massage abdomen with or without oil*
5 *Do abdominal and breathing exercises.*
6 *If necessary get up earlier in order to sit on the lavatory in a relaxed manner, at the same time each day. Continue with this even if nothing happens on the first few occasions. Try stimulating the bowel action by pressing the anus with a pad of toilet paper. It is particularly important to keep to this routine if you are taking a bulking agent; because the stool is softer you may not be getting the same painful signals.*
7 *Consider why you are so reluctant to relax your muscles. Is it fear, anger or frustration? Find someone to talk to; also use self-talk.*

Candida

1 *Kill the* Candida.
2 *Take supplements.*
3 *Keep bowel clean.*
4 *Avoid damp, mouldy environments.*
5 *Keep away from chemicals.*
6 *Get plenty of fresh air and if possible sunlight.*

Food Allergy

1 *Collect information.*
2 *See if your doctor can help.*
3 *Keep the bowel clean.*
4 *Avoid junk foods, additives, dairy produce and wheat (even before you have done your sleuthing).*
5 *Try exclusion or rotation diets.*
6 *Reactions after eating certain foods:*

a) *If your mouth swells or you have breathing difficulties, get medical help at once*

b) *If you experience flushing, palpitations, indigestion, hyperactivity or any symptom which does not need medical help and that you know is associated with what you have eaten, you could try turning the reaction off by taking:*

- *1 teaspoonful of bicarbonate of soda in warm water, or*
- *one Alka Seltzer in water, or*
- *1 gram of vitamin C, preferably in powder form. If you do use vitamin C remember it can be a stimulant.*

7 *Cool down. Research shows that food allergies are worse when you are hot. Have a cool shower, splash your face and hands with cold water or place a cold cloth on the forehead.*

8 *Try eating something else. Some people say that if they eat something they have no problems with, it seems to relieve the symptoms.*

9 *Build up your immune system by looking after your general health and taking supplements; EFAs (essential fatty acids) found in olive oil, fish oils and evening primrose oil can be helpful.*

Anxiety

1 *Slow down your thinking, speech and movements.*
2 *Do breathing exercises and relaxation in a chair for a few minutes before eating.*
3 *Don't have long gaps between meals.*
4 *Cut down on caffeine.*
5 *Investigate the calming supplements (see chapter 23).*
6 *Rest after lunch.*
7 *Take slow walks.*
8 *Do lots of self-talk.*
9 *Go to bed early.*

Agoraphobia

1 Retrain your breathing.
2 Look after your nerves generally.
3 Follow the low blood sugar pattern of eating and always have a snack before you attempt to go out.
4 Practise going out in your imagination when you are sitting in the evening; see yourself really enjoying your outing.

Depression

1 Move! Even if it feels awful, it is vital for your circulation.
2 Force yourself out of bed at the same time each day and try to this before 9 a.m.
3 Do some task each day even if you cannot finish it.
4 Eat regularly, but if you are overweight keep very low on sugar, bread, cakes, biscuits and cereals. Eat foods that will help you eliminate fluid such as garlic, onions, celery, lemon juice (unless, of course, you are sensitive to any of these).
5 Investigate supplements that stimulate (chapter 23).
6 Try to walk 20 minutes in the brightest part of the day even if it is just in the back yard or garden.
7 Do a few exercises each day; your limbs will feel like lead at first – just ignore this.
8 Breathe – if you half-breathe you will be half-dead.
9 Go to bed early. Before you go to sleep say: Every day in every way I'm getting better and better.

Alcohol Dependence

1 Hold your head up; you are not your addiction!
2 Seek help, from your doctor, friends, Alcoholics Anonymous.
3 Stop deluding yourself.
4 Keep to a strict low blood sugar eating-plan.
5 Take supplements, if possible before cutting down on alcohol.
6 Read about L-Glutamine (see pages 26–27).
7 Look after your general health.

Cigarette Dependence

1 *If you have failed many times, don't be discouraged – try again.*
2 *Keep to a very strict low blood sugar eating-plan.*
3 *Take note of all that has been said in this book about coffee.*
4 *Watch out for constipation.*
5 *Ask your doctor for help.*
6 *Start supplements four to six weeks before giving up.*
7 *Look after your general health and be patient. The misery does pass and you'll wonder how you could ever have taken such a poison.*

26

The Other You

I wake up sad and sick feeling as though I had an ulcer on my soul.
Ethan, in *The Winter of Our Discontent* by John Steinbeck

I believe that the most important part of our total well-being is the
harmony of body and soul, our spirit, higher self, inner child, God
spark or however you see it. The Divine that is in every human
being, the part of us that is with us before we incarnate and the
part of us that we return to after death. Keeping in touch with our
essence while we go through our lessons on this earth is often very
difficult. This is not about religion or how many times we go to
church. It is much wider than that. It's about our personal
relationship with the Divine, and with ourselves, no matter
how we see the Infinite – as God, Allah, Universal Energy or
Unconditional Love.

I believe that life is only the 'nursery slopes' for a life greater than
we can imagine after death. If you are sceptical about this, perhaps it
would help to read the wealth of scientific information or even popular books on near-death experiences. Overwhelmingly people who
have had this experience say that they saw a quality of light and
felt loved in a way that was totally new to them. Some sceptical

scientists say this is just some chemical reaction in the brain causing euphoria. I'm afraid this does not really 'hold water'. It does not explain how people who have been 'out of body' can give a detailed account of what has happened while they were in this state. For example the man in hospital who said the missing false teeth of the man in the end bed were behind the heating pipes and that when nurse J was in the kitchen making tea she left the fridge door open after taking out the milk. Both these statements were correct. One hospital in the south has symbols on top of the lights in the operating theatre. Patients who have been 'brought back' can describe these symbols. It has also to be said that most people who have this experience are very unwilling to 'come back' because of the joy they are experiencing. Many talk of a total acceptance and lack of fear, and how normal it feels to be with loved ones who are already there.

I believe we are here to love and learn – that is all we depart with, after all.

It is hard for me to talk about the soul without going back to the human energy field. The energy field (for which there is firm scientific evidence) surrounds the body in layers. These are sometimes called the etheric or heavenly bodies. I believe that the energy field is the 'physical' link with our soul or higher self. Observations from my own 'hands on' and Therapeutic Touch work and information from people using similar bioenergetic therapies leads me to believe that relaxation and pain relief are not the only benefits. Clients repeatedly report spiritual insights (although no reference of this possibility had been made by the therapist) and a feeling of inner strength. It is often a great surprise to people who consider they have their feet firmly on the ground. Many people report that this new awareness of themselves as spiritual beings frees them from the fear of death which they have carried for years.

My feeling is that our soul-consciousness stays in Heaven, the Universe (or whatever name we want to give it) when we are born, and through life is always concerned for our well-being and for us to complete the life-plan we chose before birth. Our spiritual progression depends on this and I believe this evolves through many lifetimes.

We hurt our soul by not loving ourselves, by not listening to our intuitive feelings or to the promptings of dreams, and by seeing the pain of life as terrible misfortunes instead of the tools we have chosen to carve out our chosen path. Salvation comes when we acknowledge the Divine in us, when we learn to forgive and love ourselves as vulnerable human beings. Only when we do this can memories be healed, can we be freed from negative emotions and treat those around us with the same gentleness.

Know Thyself, Know Thy Book-keeper

You can't cook the books of life;
The soul maintains a meticulous ledger
He'll dredge the truth from your vaults
Although your faults will not be counted.

He sits with curved back, mounted high on a stool,
Quill in hand, long-suffering, patient
And when back-taxes are due
His concern for you grows.

He gives you clues whilst you slumber
Desperate to make your numbers tally,
Toiling to keep your life-column neat, and in the black.
This is no mean feat, but He is tireless.

If you insist on resisting, you will weary first,
He cannot know defeat; eternity is on His side.
He waits for you to end the conflict,
For you to acknowledge His existence,
And for your insistence on cleaving to your personality,
Your name and frame, and for the weaving
Of insubstantial dreams to cease.

He longs for peace for you
And will use any ruse to gain a truce.
Let Him erase your fears, and take up,
With blotting paper of purest white
The tears that dim your perception.

The deception is over; take another look
Give up the fight; let Him balance your book.

In the hope that something in these pages has been of help to you
and that you will find Peace and Light in your journey through life.

Shirley Trickett

PART
THREE

Complementary

Medicine

In this section friends
who practise complementary
medicine have contributed
their approaches to digestive
problems. If you want to
investigate other alternative
therapies there are numerous
books in the shops.

Homoeopathy for Bowel Symptoms

Contributed by Beth MacEoin

The following remedies are intended as first-aid measures only. If the condition is of an ongoing, chronic variety, it will be necessary to seek professional homoeopathic help for long-term relief. In other words, treatment from a homoeopathic practitioner will deal with the predisposition to the condition. Acute or first-aid approaches will help in the short term to alleviate symptoms.

It is recommended that the most appropriate remedy should not be repeated more than three to four times daily. Once improvement has set in, discontinue the remedy. If the problem returns and the symptoms are still the same, return briefly to the same remedy, stopping again once there is further improvement. Do not persevere with a remedy which is not helping in the hope it will eventually take effect. This is an indication that the choice is incorrect, and a more appropriate prescription is needed.

Generally speaking, if it is necessary to repeat the indicated remedy for a few days in succession, professional help should be sought to deal with the condition more effectively. On the other hand, the relief gained from judicious homoeopathic prescribing for a day or so can be enormous.

The following list of conditions and appropriate remedies is intended only as a rough guide. More information may be obtained from books such as: *How to Use Homoeopathy Effectively*, Christopher Hammond (Carotas Healthcare, 1988); *Everybody's Guide to Homoeopathic Remedies*, Cummings and Ullman (Gollancz, 1984); *Homoeopathic Medicine at Home*, Panos and Heimlich (Corgi, 1984) and *The Family Guide to Homoeopathy*, Dr Andrew Lockie (Elm Tree Books, 1988).

For further information and advice on choosing a practitioner, contact the Society of Homoeopaths, 2 Artizan Road, Northampton, NN1 4HU, Telephone 01604 621400.

Flatulence

As with any conditions affecting the digestive tract, dietary indiscretions should be rectified – this may be enough to improve the problem dramatically. Any of the following remedies should bring fast relief provided the picture fits. They are intended as aids to short-term relief only. As in the case of antacids, regular dosing with homoeopathic remedies is not recommended.

Carbo Veg.

Someone needing *Carbo Veg.* may experience bloating and distension in the abdominal regions which is much worse after eating even the smallest quantity of food. Distension is so bad that any pressure around the waist causes discomfort, and waistbands must be loosened. Relief is obtained from passing wind in either direction. There is likely to be a total aversion to any kind of food, especially meat, fatty foods and milk. The stomach is likely to feel very heavy after eating due to slowness of digestion. The person needing *Carbo Veg.* will often feel much better for exposure to fresh air and may generally feel much worse for being in a stuffy atmosphere.

Pulsatilla

Someone needing *Pulsatilla* may complain that their mouth feels dry, but they are not thirsty. This sensation may follow eating an overly fatty meal. The tongue may be coated with a thick white or yellow deposit, while there may be a stone-like sensation in the stomach. Accompanying nausea may be aggravated by warm liquids and relieved by cold drinks. There may be a bad taste in the mouth on waking, and the taste of food previously eaten may come up with burping – this may remain in the mouth for a long time. Pain of flatulence is made worse by the jarring of a misstep while walking. Generally may feel worse resting and better for a gentle motion. Although chilly, may desire fresh air.

Nux Vomica

Digestive disturbance following overindulgence in rich food, alcohol, or smoking. Disturbance may also be related to toxicity from overuse of drugs such as painkillers or laxatives, or lack of sleep from burning the candle at both ends. Flatulence is likely to be related to constipation, which may be habitual as a result of bad eating habits. Food lies in the stomach feeling like a heavy knot and may give rise to hiccups. Burps taste sour and are difficult to bring up. The person needing *Nux Vomica* may feel hungry but also averse to food at the same time. Colicky pain in the abdomen is relieved once a bowel movement has been achieved.

Lycopodium

Even after a little food has been eaten, there may be an uncomfortable sensation of fullness in the stomach or abdomen leading to distension, rumblings and gurglings. Unlike the person requiring *Carbo Veg.* for flatulence, the person needing *Lycopodium* will not get any relief from the passage of wind in either direction. Flatulence may be relieved by taking hot drinks (the opposite of *Pulsatilla*. Burning sensation with burping which settles in the throat. Digestive problems may be linked with anxiety symptoms – especially anticipatory anxiety before an important event.

Constipation

As with the preceding section, the following remedies are intended for short-term use only. It is generally not helpful to exchange regular doses of laxatives for regular doses of the appropriate homoeopathic remedy, since underlying causes must be dealt with, rather than being dependent on medication for the regulation of symptoms.

Nux Vomica

Often indicated for people who have become dependent on regular doses of laxatives connected to a busy sedentary lifestyle. The stool may be described as 'bashful' because of its tendency to incomplete evacuation. Those needing *Nux Vomica* are likely to experience a sensation of never quite having completed a bowel motion – it often feels as though something has been left behind. There may be a strong urge for a bowel movement, but however much straining is done, nothing seems to happen. There may also be a residual burning sensation in the rectum once the bowels have acted. Irritability and physical and mental oversensitivity are likely to accompany the problem.

Bryonia

Unlike the *Nux Vomica* picture, those needing *Bryonia* are unlikely to feel any desire to move their bowels. Because of poor internal secretions, once a stool is passed, it is accompanied with much difficulty, and appears large, dry and dark as though burnt. There may be a strong sense of thirst for cold water in large quantities. As with *Nux Vomica*, there may be marked irritability and headache.

Alumina

Even a soft stool is expressed with difficulty due to lack of tone of the rectum. No inclination to try to pass a stool, but when a motion is obtained, it is likely to be soft and sticky, or hard and knotted. There may also be itching and burning at the anus.

Graphites

Soreness and itching of the anus with possible aching after passing a stool. Several days may go by without urging, but when a motion is achieved, it is likely to consist of small, rounded pellets covered with shreds of mucus. There may be a tendency to anal fissure which causes great pain on passage of a stool. Persons needing Graphites may have a tendency to be overweight and chilly.

Diarrhoea

Arsenicum Album

Pains are burning in character and accompanied by fearfulness, anxiety and restlessness. Chilliness will accompany digestive upsets and symptoms may be markedly worse at night on both physical and mental levels. Eating will generally aggravate the problem, while sips of liquid and warmth in general are helpful. Diarrhoea will be violent, watery, burning, very offensive, and may smell putrid. The person displaying *Arsenicum* symptoms will be quickly prostrated by their condition, and often show a marked need for company and sympathy.

Veratrum Album

More sweaty with diarrhoea than the person needing *Arsenicum*. After a bout of diarrhoea the sufferer feels cold, clammy, and about to collapse. The pain accompanying the diarrhoea forces the person to bend double. Diarrhoea is likely to be copious and may be colourless. During and after a bout of diarrhoea, the person may look bluish-white and perspire all over the body in a cold sweat. Prostration will be extreme with very sudden onset. During the bout of diarrhoea there may be an unquenchable thirst for cold drinks. Diarrhoea may follow on from prolonged exposure to stress or a sudden fright.

Podophyllum

Diarrhoea very profuse and offensive. Large quantities are passed with each bowel movement which happens with terrific frequency. Motions are likely to be completely liquid and may be a greenish-yellow in colour. Diarrhoea may be painless, or cramping pains may come on before, or during the passage of fluid which is squirted out with force and noise. Cramps are relieved by warm applications and bending double. Colicky pains may continue for some time after the diarrhoea has passed.

Pulsatilla

Diarrhoea that is aggravated by a perpetually over-rich, fatty diet. Physical symptoms include: changeable pain with changeable location, and dissimilarity between bowel movements, no two of which look alike. Queasiness and indigestion may accompany the diarrhoea, while eating results in a feeling of heaviness. The mouth will be dry, but the person needing *Pulsatilla* will be thirstless. Diarrhoea is aggravated by being over-warm and drinking warm liquids, and it may be very bad at night. There is much belching and bloating, and constipation may alternate with diarrhoea. Weepiness and sadness may accompany the latter, or there will be changeability of moods from one phase to another. Sympathy is likely to be strongly appreciated. The patient responds well to fresh air or gentle motion.

Beth MacEoin B.A. (Swansea), B.A. (Newcastle), M.N.C.H.M.

Therapeutic Massage

Contributed by Mandy Wilkinson

Massage is one of the most ancient and universal of the healing arts. For thousands of years some form of massage or laying on of hands has been used to heal and relieve pain, although the value of massage is often underestimated in today's 'sophisticated' world.

Therapeutic massage is the art of restoring vitality, reducing muscular tension, and increasing health and well-being by manipulating the soft body tissues with the hands. By relaxing the body, massage can relieve both physical *and* mental tension, combating the overall effects of stress which are at the root of all illness. It can thus be beneficial for a wide variety of symptoms. Taut, painful muscles are loosened and relaxed. The circulation of blood and lymph is stimulated, resulting in the expulsion of toxins from the body, and the eventual restoration of balanced tone in the muscles and greater freedom in the joints. As muscles relax and circulation can function more efficiently, digestion and elimination, breathing and posture all improve as a result.

As the body starts to change and heal with regular massage, feelings of depression, anxiety, fear or irritability – so often the side-effects of chronic patterns of tension – may eventually begin to lift. Thus, massage is beneficial not just for the body, but also for the mental and emotional aspects of a person. As such it is an important holistic therapy, much more than just a 'luxury', as it is often seen, or a way of treating only sports injuries.

Mandy Wilkinson
(Practitioner of therapeutic massage and yoga teacher)

29

Colonic Irrigation

Contributed by Andrea Warwick

Colonic lavage was first recorded in 1500 BC in the ancient
Egyptian document, *Ebers Papyrus*, which dealt with the practice
of medicine. The enemas were described as the infusion of aqueous
substances in to the large intestine through the anus. In the fourth
and fifth centuries BC, Hippocrates recorded using enemas for fever
therapy and in the second century AD Galen recognized and used
enemas. In AD 1600 Paré offered the distinction between colonic
irrigation and the popular enema therapy of that time.

Ideally we should eliminate after every meal, two or three times a
day. Most people consider themselves in good working order if they
have one bowel movement a day and many more do not even
achieve that amount of regularity. When the colon is clean and
healthy we experience a feeling of well-being. The colon is in
effect the sewage system of the body and like any rubbish bin it is
susceptible to stagnations and the formation of decay and poisonous
substances. It therefore needs special care to keep it clean from
putrefaction. When this does not happen, the decay is not limited
to the site of origin. It spreads rapidly to other organs, causing
auto-intoxication or self-poisoning.

This poisoning affects all of the body's tissues and can take many forms. If the poisoning is in the brain and nervous system it makes us depressed and irritable. If in the heart, we become weak and lack energy. In the lungs it can make us breathless and cause halitosis (bad breath), and in the stomach, the toxins cause bloating. When these toxins are found in the blood and lymph system we are sure to have a sallow, spotty and unclean looking skin and if they back up to the glands, we feel tired, lacking enthusiasm, sex drive and look old beyond our years.

The gradual spread of this toxaemia can lead to all kinds of stomach ulcers, cancers, colitis, diverticulitis, gall bladder inflammation, infection of the gums, tooth decay, fatty degeneration of the heart, abnormal blood pressure, arteriosclerosis, headaches, neuralgia, arthritis and so on – the list is endless.

The colon is the largest perpetrator of disease of any organ of the body. It is said to be the initiator of 80 per cent of all critical illnesses. Many people go around permanently constipated, and because they know no different, take headaches, lethargy and general depletion for granted. They simply do not remember what it is like to have a healthy colon and a feeling of well-being.

Constipation occurs when any waste material is retained by the colon. Instead of their natural smooth state, the walls of the colon become encrusted with this accumulated faecal matter which is similar to hard black rubber; it builds up year after year. Since the encrusted faeces form a barrier, the colon is unable to absorb or eliminate properly. The muscles cannot move to make the wave-like actions to move waste along. Toxins from fermentation, putrefaction and wastes from the blood stream which should normally be drawn through the colon and eliminated are reabsorbed by the body along with incompletely digested food. Remember if you suffer regular diarrhoea you are as constipated as the person who does not eliminate regularly. A loose stool can rush through and still leave the old residue on the walls of the bowel. Good health is as much a function of how we eliminate from our bodies as to as what we take in. Yet $50 million in annual laxative sales in the United States indicates that elimination is a problem for many people. At least five million people in the United Kingdom suffer from constipation, colitis, diverticulitis, and ileitis and 200,000 each year have a colostomy. Cancer of the colon is second only to heart disease as the most common cause of death in the United Kingdom. This need not be so.

Edible Intake

Improper diet, insufficient exercise, stress, overeating and ignoring the call of nature can all lead to bowel problems. Fibre-rich food is not the complete answer. Some people eat lots of bran (usually wheat bran, and 30 per cent of people are wheat intolerant); wheat scours the delicate lining of the bowel, and if the person is constipated it will make the condition worse by achieving nothing other than an irritable bowel and lots of flatulence.

Fibre is the bit that is left behind once the food is digested. It is considered good for us because it helps to provide bulk to otherwise watery wastes in the colon, and absorbs toxicity; but it is no good if the colon is already prone to blockage. Like the rest of the waste, some types of fibre will become stagnant and add to the congestion.

Better alternatives to bran are roughage from other vegetable bases, such as oats and rice. These tend not to be so abrasive and to swell into a mucilaginous gel which acts as a gentle detoxifier.

One common sign of trouble, dense sticky bowel movements, indicates an excess of mucus in the system. This is usually the product of mucus-producing foods such as dairy products, flour and meat. Meat is extremely contaminating to the bowel and prone to putrefaction, and in a short time creates a great strain on the elimination system.

Mucus stools are the most difficult to eliminate. They leave behind the glue-like coating on the wall of the colon which accumulates layer upon layer into a hard rubbery crust. This is carried for the duration of the person's life as a toxic burden.

Balancing the Microbes

Microbes sound like another unmentionable, but in fact they are essential to our well-being. The colon contains between 3 and 4 lbs of micro-organisms. There are about 400 varieties; most of which are fungi, along with viruses, bacteria and many others. Normally they function together in friendly co-existence, completing the digestion, producing vitamins and controlling infection, but this balance is fragile and easily upset. For example sudden exposure to the alkaline medium of the caecum causes yeasts to proliferate. Long-term constipation, harsh laxatives and any course of antibiotics or drugs will destroy the balance. When undesirable bacteria take the upper hand, the gut is in trouble, we may experience stomach pains and bloating, excess gas, headaches, allergies and skin conditions. This is the reason why upset stomachs often go hand in hand with courses of antibiotics. The proliferation of *Candida Albicans* and similar moulds and yeasts can give rise to whole sets of symptoms.

What is Colonic Hydrotherapy?

Colonic Hydrotherapy or Irrigation may sound a far-fetched answer to all these problems but it is really no more than an internal bath, helping to cleanse the colon of poisons, gas and accumulated matter. Unlike an enema it does not involve the retention of water. Just a steady flow in and out, stimulating the colon to recover its natural shape, tone and peristaltic wave action. It also reaches along the intestines further than an enema.

A series of four to eight colonics is recommended at first, depending on the patient's circumstances. Have no fear – colonic irrigation is a pleasant experience involving neither embarrassment nor discomfort. Some patients have been known to doze off during treatment.

The patient lies on a couch next to a temperature controlled input tank, and a triple-sterilized speculum is gently inserted into the rectum. The water temperature and pressure are carefully monitored by the therapist. Filtered water flows into the colon via a small tube and out through another tube called the evacuation tube. The colon will start to feel full, then the water is released carrying with it impacted faeces and mucus. As the waters flows out of the colon the therapist gently massages the abdomen to assist the release of its contents. The therapist can watch the contents being discharged through inspection of the evacuation tube. The system is completely closed so there is no odour or external contact with the water. The whole process takes around half an hour and the patient is well covered throughout the treatment – modesty is given top priority.

Afterwards it is quite normal to have the urge to visit the toilet especially on your first session, after which you will feel extremely empty. After a series of treatments a lactobacillus implant is usually given via the rectum to replace any bacteria that have been washed out.

The best thing about colonic treatment is how good you feel afterwards. There will be other signs too of the beneficial effects, a pinker complexion, brighter eyes and more energy. A series of colonics is sometimes necessary to dislodge hardened waste. It is most effective when employed in combination with exercise and proper diet of non-mucus producing foods.

Certain herbs also help to loosen and dislodge accumulated encrusted material. Once the colon is clean maintenance is important – good diet and self-help to keep the bowel running smoothly and single colonic treatments are desirable two to four times per year. They are a first-class spring clean. A good time is the change of the seasons, when the diet and exercise often change. Another ideal time is before, during and after a fast to hasten the removal of toxic waste. If you decide to change your diet to a more healthy style, what better way than to have a good clean out in order to start your new eating programme afresh? Irrigation is also beneficial during the cold and flu season. Nutritional and dietary counselling is given to assist the client in maintaining a healthy colon.

By cleansing the colon of impacted and putrefactive faecal matter, colonic irrigation relieves the system of a variety of disturbances, including fatigue, gas, headaches, irritability, skin problems, cold hands and feet, lethargy, constipation (of course) as well as chronic diarrhoea, colitis, diverticulitis, Crohn's disease and many more. With colonic irrigation, your sense of well-being is often dramatically improved. The body can again take nourishment from food and defend itself against disease. Natural peristalsis, tone and regularity are restored and many serious diseases may be averted through this gentle, sterile and scientific technique. Colonic irrigation is a key factor in restoration of the sparkling health we all can, and should have.

Andrea Warwick, RCT-MCIA

For further information regarding treatments write to:

Andrea Warwick, RCT-MCIA
Northern Natural Therapies
41 Teesway
Neasham
Darlington DL2 1QT

Edward Bryce RCT-MCIA, Corinne Bryce RCT-MCIA
Fife Natural Therapies
178 Pitcorthie Drive
Dunfermline
Fife KY11 5DF

Colonic International Association
26 Sea Road
Boscombe
Bournemouth
Dorset BH5 1DF

30

Reflexology

Contributed by Andrea Warwick

Reflexology has been used for five thousand years in China and in AD 1027 it is recorded as having been used as an energy balancing procedure. It is a form of holistic healing (taken from the Greek word *holos* meaning 'whole') and as with any holistic principle,

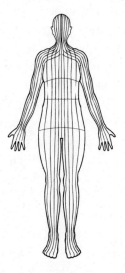

Fig. 7. Reflexology zones

three aspects must be involved in order to achieve a feeling of balance and well being, the mind, the body, and the spirit.

In the early 1900s an American, Dr William Fitzgerald, discovered that there are ten electrical currents running through the body from the top of the head to the toes in line with the toes and fingers. Each area covered by a current is called a zone and there are five zones of each side of the body. All the organs, glands and nervous systems fall within these zones. Crystalline deposits form around the nerve endings preventing the electrical contact of the nerves from earthing via the feet and hands. By applying pressure to the nerve endings the crystalline deposits can be broken up and the nerves are able to 'earth', balance and order can be restored and a smooth flow of vibratory energy spreads throughout the body.

During the 1930s, zone therapist Eunice Ingham began to feel that the feet specifically could be used for therapy because of their highly sensitive nature. She charted the feet in relation to the zones and the effects they had on the rest of the anatomy until she finally evolved a map of the feet reflecting the entire body, all parts of the body being related to specific areas, called reflexes, on the hands and feet. Sensitivity in a specific part of the foot is a signal that there is congestion or tension in that zone. By applying direct alternating pressure on the foot, therapeutic benefits are set in motion throughout the entire zonal area. Zone therapy is the basis of foot reflexology, and has now become a very refined system.

The feet resemble the human body, the left foot relating to the left side of the head and body and the right foot relating to the right side of the head and body. If you place both feet together in front of you, you will see that each big toe represents half the head and neck, the ball of the big toe representing the head and the stem of the big toe represents the neck. The spine runs down the inside of each foot, the shoulder joints occur on the outside of the feet just below the little toe. On the outside of the foot roughly halfway down is a protruding bone; if you draw an imaginary line across the sole of the foot, that represents the waistline. Organs found in the body above the waistline have reflexes above this line on the foot and organs below the waistline have reflexes between this line and the heel. So it can be seen that reflexology is a science that deals with the principle that there are reflexes in the feet relative to each and every organ, function and part of the body.

The approach of reflexology is to treat the individual as a whole in order to create a better harmony between the mind, the body, and the emotions, thereby helping to restore some of the lost energy and re-establish a more positive attitude towards the world. Reflexology relaxes tension, improves nerve and blood supply and restores balance to the body. If you have a long standing disorder that does not seem to have been helped by orthodox medical treatment, then give reflexology a try. It is a therapy that is safe and also very effective, but remember if your disorder has been with you for a long time it cannot be rectified overnight. Your body has the ability to heal itself once the process has been set in motion.

It is medically accepted that 75 per cent of all disease is caused by stress, and the greatest benefit you can receive from reflexology is relaxation. It has a dynamic effect on the body in its ability to relieve stress and tension. As a means of diagnosis reflexology is quick and accurate. By testing the reflexes of the feet, the degree of tenderness gives an accurate indication of any area that is out of balance. Effective results are to be found even after two or three treatments. Reflexology creates a feeling of well-being, enabling those suffering from anxiety states some respite from their symptoms.

What Happens at a Consultation

Having removed the shoes and stockings and been comfortably seated with feet raised, diagnosis is carried out by feeling the hands or feet and noting the position of tender reflex areas. The hands have the same reflex areas as the feet. A case history may then be taken.

Treatment consists of compressing and massaging the foot as a whole paying particular attention to the tender areas to break down the crystalline deposits and free the energy flow. No limit can be set as to the number of treatments necessary; this varies according to the type of disorder and whether it is longstanding or recent.

For further information regarding treatment write to:

Andrea Warwick, Natural Health Therapist
Northern Natural Therapies
41 Teesway
Neasham
Darlington DL2 1QT

For details of training courses write to:

The British Reflexology Association
Monks Orchard
Whitbourne
Worcester WR6 5RB

Ann Gillanders
The Holistic Healing Centre
92 Sheering Road
Old Harlow
Essex CM17 0JT

31

Shiatsu

Contributed by Paul Lambeth

Shiatsu is a Japanese word literally translated as 'finger pressure'. It developed from traditional oriental massage practised in the home by the 'barefoot doctors' over 3,000 years ago, and today its evolution continues to adapt to our constantly changing lifestyles.

Shiatsu is based upon an understanding of the human body as a system of energy. Just as when we place a magnet below a piece of paper with iron filings on top we see a pattern expressing the magnetic energy field, so too there is order to the electromagnetic field of the human body. This energy circulates through our body in channels called meridians, activating and charging our internal organs and their functions.

The activities of modern life distort our pattern of energy and these channels become blocked and imbalanced, affecting us both physically and emotionally. During shiatsu hands and thumbs are applied with varying degrees of pressure and the body may be stretched or kneaded so that areas of tension are relaxed, and points of weakness revitalized. This stimulates and harmonizes the flow of our energy, and the body's natural healing force is awakened to restore well-being. Relief can be gained from such symptoms are back pain, stress, asthma, stiffness, headaches, insomnia and so on.

Pressure on specific points not only releases hormones including natural pain-killers, but also improves the circulation of blood lymph and affects the nervous system. Receiving shiatsu is a special experience which is both relaxing and rejuvenating. How often you have shiatsu will depend upon your own personal needs and goals. Whether for instance you wish to maintain or regain your health, and upon your body's individual self healing capacity.

Unlike Western massage the receiver remains fully clothed throughout. As a natural therapy shiatsu is most effective when you wear comfortable clothing of natural fibres, such as a cotton track suit.

Many physical complaints are accompanied by some psychological conditions, so in addition to physical relief, shiatsu will also affect these. For instance with disorders of the colon we often feel depressed and lacking initiative and openness; we withhold our emotions; or we may feel stress in our shoulders, caused by short shallow breathing.

Since it is our day-to-day activities which determine the quality of our health, the experienced shiatsu practitioner will give you suggestions on aspects of your lifestyle such as diet, physical activity, breathing patterns and relaxation techniques. Some are able to give you specific macrobiotic dietary advice. Such suggestions will enable you to make positive changes and take greater responsibility for your own health.

Exercises to Strengthen the Digestive System

1. Chewing

Chew all your food until it becomes liquid (at least 50 times per mouthful). Chewing is the very beginning of the digestive process; if we fail to fulfil this simple task we can cause havoc to the remainder of the digestive system.

Unfortunately many people eat on the run, or while preoccupied with other things and ingest them along with the food inflicting them on the digestive systems and perpetuating them. If we chew thoroughly we break this chain, as chewing causes us to slow down, creating a more harmonious eating experience, stress-free digestion and a happier digestive system.

Please remember to chew very well, especially if you have a tendency to overeat.

2. Exercise

Keeping physically active does not necessarily mean jogging or going to the gym. Each type of physical activity has a different effect upon our physical and mental state.

Long walks are especially recommended as is 'constructive exercise', like cleaning the house. House-cleaning not only gives you the opportunity to stretch your body in many ways as vigorously as you wish, but also creates order in your immediate external environment, and so in your body and your mind. Ever tried thinking clearly in a chaotic room?

We tend to choose leisure activities that compound our nature, so that a more physically aggressive person will take up some vigorous sport, whereas someone who is inclined to daydream will gravitate towards meditation. However, very often the more physically oriented person would benefit from meditation, just as the person leading a more sedentary life would benefit from something more vigorous. Choose some activity that complements and harmonizes your nature.

3. Deep Breathing

1   *Lie flat on your back with one hand on top of the other, the palm resting on your lower abdomen. Exhale thoroughly through your open mouth then close your mouth and inhale through your nose. As the breath goes in, let it take your attention to your lower abdomen, while your belly rises, your hands also rise. Hold the breath for at least 10 seconds then exhale so that your belly becomes flat and your hands once again fall.*

Continue relaxed deep breathing focusing on sending the breath deep into your lower abdomen and on the rise and fall of your hands. If you become aware of any tension do exercise (2) then repeat deep breathing.

2 Stand with feet shoulder-width apart, and with the palm of one hand on top of the other rub in a clockwise motion around the abdominal area. Do this for one minute.

3 Standing with feet shoulder-width apart and hands resting on your hips, rotate your hips. Try and make the centre of the movement as low as possible. First in one direction for a minute then reverse.

4 With feet flat on the floor and hands linked behind the head adopt a crouched position. Bounce up and down and try to squat as deeply as possible.

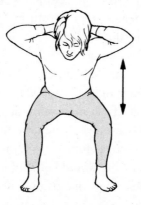

Then continue bobbing up and down and describe a circular motion, first one way and then the other.

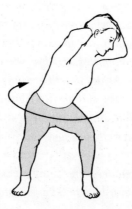

5   *Crouch down with hands linked together on top of your head.*

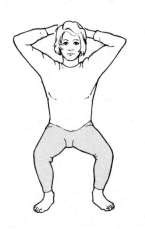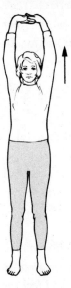

   Breathe in and stand up on tiptoes, turning your hands over so that the palms face upward. Stretch as high as you can, then exhale and stretch again before returning to your original position. Repeat 10 times.

6   *Standing with feet shoulder-width apart swing your arms around from one side to the other towards the back to twist your spine.*

   Then making two light fists, continue swinging but as you swing to the left and exhale, bang your lower back with your left fist at the same time as banging your lower abdomen with your right fist. As you swing to the right you exhale while banging your lower back with your right fist and lower abdomen with your left fist. Make this a smooth rhythmic motion.

7   *When digestive disorders are present we often experience tension in the shoulders and lower back. To relax the shoulders rotate the arms in each direction. Bunch your shoulders up towards your ears trying to make as much tension as possible then quickly release and feel them relax.*

   To loosen the lower back lie on the floor with your hands behind your head and bring your feet up to where your knees were. Drop your knees down to either side.

As you bring your feet further towards your body you
experience the stretch higher in your back.

8   *Lie on the floor on your back with your arms at the side and*
your feet together, toes pointing upward.

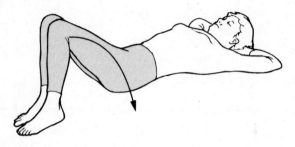

Raise your feet a few inches from the floor and hold for
20 seconds or so as you breathe deeply and relax. Lower your
feet and feel the small of your back relax and sink lower into
the floor.

Paul Lambeth has a shiatsu practice in the north of England, and
teaches for the Kushi Institute and Community Health Foundation
in London.

Enquiries to:
Paul Lambeth   Community Health Foundation
Albert Cottage   188 Old Street
Townhead   London EC1U 9BP
Alston   0171 251 4076
Cumbria CA9 3SL

The Shiatsu Society
19 Langside Park
Kilbarchan
Renfrewshire PA10 2EP

32

Aromatherapy

Contributed by Carole Cunningham I.P.T.I.

Aromatherapy is the use of essential oils as a form of health care. Nowadays as people are becoming more aware of environmental pollution and chemical hazards, they are searching for natural remedies to promote their health and well-being. By using aromatherapy we can help ourselves to restore the energy lost from our own physical exertion, and from the effects of the age in which we live.

Essential oils are natural extracts from plants, fruit, wood and resins. In their purest form, they are molecular substances that carry the characteristic fragrance of the source from which they have been extracted. They have been described as having hormonal qualities that hold the life force from each living substance whence they derive.

Thousands of years ago the Egyptians used aromatic oils to add to their baths, and for centuries priests burned Frankincense in religious ceremonies to produce spiritual calmness. Our not so distant ancestors used herbs in the form of pomanders to protect themselves from infection, and elderly ladies were calmed and refreshed by Lavender water if they succumbed to an attack of 'the vapours'.

The knowledge of the wider use of essential oils was lost for several hundred years, and more recently, about 30 years ago, it was brought over to England from France by a woman called Madame Maury, who had promoted its valuable use in skin care. As it was discovered that essential oils absorb through the fatty tissue beneath the skin, they were combined with vegetable oils and used in the form of a massage treatment, which produced a regenerative and healing effect on the whole body.

The term aromatherapy was used to describe this treatment, and from that point a system of healing was initiated which was slowly to become more widely recognized.

Although there are many sceptics who refuse to accept a therapy which has not been scientifically proven, there is no doubt that most people under stress react favourably to this form of therapy. It is therefore being introduced into some hospitals as part of the patient care programme, and student nurses are being educated in the techniques of therapeutic touch. More recently public awareness has been increased through the media, and the essential oil industry is beginning to boom.

My own interest in aromatherapy began about five years ago, when I read an article in a health magazine. I decided to experiment with Lavender and Neroli as massage oils for relaxation in my neck and shoulders. Following a neck injury I often felt discomfort from muscle spasm, and found that the gentle relaxation that the oils produced freed me from pain and tension in that area. Not only was the pain relieved, but my whole body felt better for having experienced the process. At that time I searched to find an aromatherapist who could treat me, but there was no one practising within my area, so it was then that I made the decision to train to become an aromatherapist.

I am a qualified nurse, and having worked in hospital for many years in both the general and psychiatric field, I have always been concerned that patients have been offered tranquillizers and analgesics far too frequently in order to suppress their tensions. Increased tension in muscles caused through pain, worry, or strenuous activity that the body is unable to handle, is stored beneath the surface, unable to be easily released. This creates a vicious cycle which ultimately causes lowered morale through anxiety, and as our energy levels decrease, can lead to depression and serious forms of ill health.

As many physical disorders are related to stress, it is necessary to work on this angle in order to induce general healing. As one develops a freedom from tension, it is easier for us to be more aware of our lifestyle and the frustrations and causes which have led to our symptoms. We all have a part in our bodies which holds a weak point, and for many of us the digestive tract is the part that suffers. At the first sign of stress, our diaphragm tightens, immediately restricting our normal breathing pattern, causing us to feel tense and anxious. This in turn releases the mechanisms which come into play as our 'fight or flight' response. During this process, large amounts of adrenaline are released into our circulatory system. Adrenaline is a chemical which is released into our bloodstream at times of stress, in order to increase energy levels into our muscles to give us the strength to run away from a fearful situation, or to stay and attack. If we do not do either, our muscles tend to stay in this state of tension as the process is repeated, and this in turn evokes other responses. The nerves in our digestive tract become exposed to our anxieties and behave in a disorderly manner. This causes pain, loss of appetite and digestive upsets, which in turn lead to more anxiety. The food we eat may not be fully absorbed, we feel bloated and uncomfortable, and again the tension increases.

The vicious cycle, once established, is difficult to break, unless we do something to help our bodies to relax, and recognize what we can do to help ourselves. As a natural health care practitioner, I instruct my patients how to achieve full body relaxation, which allows each individual to learn to control this build up of tension. Relaxation therapy, combined with aromatherapy treatments, and a back up of self-help at home, is a useful aid in helping the body to respond to the demands of stress.

A qualified aromatherapist will begin a consultation by taking a case history from the patient they are treating. The person's lifestyle and full medical history are taken into account in order to select the correct oils suitable for an individual treatment. The most important factor to be considered, as there are many oils to choose from in most cases, is that the person being treated appreciates and enjoys the fragrance being used. Essential oils are volatile substances, and during the evaporation process are absorbed by our sense of smell to reach various parts of the brain. This triggers off a chemical reaction in glands and organs throughout the body. Fragrances can evoke memories and produce emotional waves that nurture and calm our basic instincts.

Although treatment by a qualified therapist is obviously most beneficial, there is no reason why we cannot treat ourselves, or find a partner to help. Providing the technique used is simple and relaxing, intuitive massage by another caring person can help considerably.

Essential oils should only be blended for massage purposes by a qualified aromatherapist as they are highly potent substances.

For the lay person to use on adults only there are many relaxing formulations which are blended in a carrier oil base. It is important to note that if these are used on elderly people they should be diluted to half strength in a suitable carrier oil such as cosmetically refined soyabean oil or avocado oil.

Essential oils should always be diluted for use in massage in a carrier oil base and should never be taken internally.

A gentle back massage releases muscular tension, which is an important step in tackling any physical problem, and formulations which include sandalwood, ylang ylang, lavender and neroli all have calming and relaxing qualities which are good for this purpose.

Before you begin a massage treatment, ensure that the room you are using is warm, and that you have sufficient towels to place beneath you, and to cover the areas that are not being exposed to massage treatment.

When I give someone a back massage, I always smooth a little of the substance being used on to the person's forearm, so as they lie face downwards they have the benefit of inhaling the fragrance at the same time. Some people enjoy the sound of soft music playing in the background, and the light in the room should be gentle and unobtrusive. Any disturbance from outside noise and interruptions should be avoided so that the whole atmosphere is calm and receptive to the treatment.

Essential oils can be used in the bath, either blended with a carrier oil, or in their pure concentrated form. Six drops in the bath water should provide adequate fragrance for a relaxing bath. Ensure that you agitate the water well before you sit down, as the oils can sink to the bottom of the bath, and in the event of direct contact may cause skin sensitivity. Peppermint and citrus oils should be used with caution for this same purpose.

Oil burners can create an interesting fragrance in your home environment. As all the oils contain antiseptic qualities, they make useful air fresheners. Frankincense and Bergamot can calm and uplift our senses. In this way you can experiment with the use of essential oils, and through your own intuition discover ways of alleviating your stresses and enhancing your well-being.

Carole Cunningham R.G.N. (Diploma in Clinical Aromatherapy) works as practice nurse for Dr Damien Downing and practises aromatherapy at his clinic in York.

Enquiries to:
Nutrition Associates
Galtres House
Lysander Close
Clifton Moorgate
York YO3 0XB

Laburnum Cottage
Main Street
Melbourne
York YO4 4QQ

Useful Addresses

IBS Network
c/o Centre for Human Nutrition
Northern General Hospital
Sheffield S5 7AU

Run by IBS sufferers for IBS sufferers.

Biolab Medical Unit
9 Weymouth St
London W1N 3FF

New Nutrition
Woodlands
London Road, Battle
East Sussex TN33 0LP
(01424) 774103

Many people are now seeking natural ways to cleanse the digestive
system from the effects of drugs and careless eating habits and also
to build up the nervous system and immune system with vitamins
and minerals. It is essential to have expert advice on this. New

Nutrition is staffed by experienced nutritionists. Advice is available via a Natural Health Hot Line, the Health Letter Service, the computer assisted CARE programme, and personal nutrition consultants. Offer seminars on nutrition, special diets, natural health and skin care. Membership costs £5 per year (at the time of writing) and includes telephone advice on which supplements to order and a magazine three times a year. There is a charge of £3 if you write for advice on your health problems.

The Society for the Promotion of Nutritional Therapy
PO Box 47
Heathfield
East Sussex TN21 8ZX

Send SAE for list of nutritionists in your area

Higher Nature
Burwash Common
East Sussex TN19 7LX
Mail order (01435) 882880
Fax (01435) 883720
Team of qualified nutritionists able to give advice: (01435) 883964

Higher Nature is dedicated to providing a comprehensive nutritional service. The quality of supplements is excellent, and the 'Nutrition and Beyond' offprints are well worth the 30-pence price (at the time of writing). Higher Nature makes regular contributions of supplements and money to refugees and those in nutritional need. They also have an outstanding range of skin care products. Reliable testing for *Candida* and allergies (Annemarie Borlind).

Biocare Ltd
54 Northfield Road
Norton
Birmingham B30 1JH
(0121) 433 3727

Suppliers of a wide range of high-quality nutritional products.

Nutrition Associates
Galtres House
Lysander Close
Clifton Moorgate
York YO3 OXB
(01904) 691591

A medical practice dealing with all nutritional problems. A variety
of treatments available including Full-Spectrum Light Therapy.
Information on full-spectrum lighting for the home and workplace.

The Complete Hormone Clinic
Dr Andrew Wright
57 Chorley New Road
Bolton
Lancs BL1 4QR
(01204) 366101

Dr Wright is trained in orthodox and complementary medicine. He
has a great interest in chronic fatigue, *Candida* and allergies.

Labscan
Biomedical Screening Service
Silver Birches
Private Road
Rodborough Common
Stroud
Glos GL5 5BY
(01435) 873446/873668
Fax (01435) 878588

Labscan is an independent laboratory established to provide a
non-invasive, simple to use, comprehensive diagnostic service for
nutritionists and other practitioners who wish to determine the
ecological status of their patient's intestinal tract.

Michael Franklin
1 Squitchey Lane
Apartment 4
Oxford OX2 7LB
(01865) 511357

Mr Franklin is a trained nutritionist with a special interest in IBS, chronic fatigue, *Candida* and allergies.

The Radionics Association
Goose Green
Deddington
Nr Banbury OX15 0SZ

I can personally recommend (as can many of my clients and readers) this little-known alternative approach. It is useful in a wide variety of conditions. For a practitioner in your area, contact above address.

Mrs D Frankish, Radionics Practitioner
4 Relton Terrace
Monkseaton
Whitely Bay
Tyne and Wear NE25 8DY

Health Interlink
(01582) 794094

Reasonably priced hair analysis for vitamin and mineral status.

Action Against Allergy (Amelia Hill)
43 The Downs
London SW20 8HG

AAA (Action Against Allergy) provides an information service on all aspects of allergy and allergy-related illness, which is free to everyone. Supporting members get a Newsletter three times a year and a postal lending library service. AAA can supply GPs with the names and addresses of specialist allergy doctors. It also has a talk-line network which puts sufferers in contact with others through the NHS and initiates and supports research. Please enclose SAE (9" x 6") for further information.

National Association of Colitis and Crohn's Disease
98A London Road
St Albans, Herts AL1 1NX

National Society for Research into Allergy
PO Box 45, Hinckley
Leicestershire LE10 1JY

Cirrus Associates
Food and Environmental Consultancy
Little Hintock
Kington Magna
Gillingham, Dorset SP8 5EW
(01747) 838165

A wide range of products including VDU screen protectors, allergy-safe kettles and cooking appliances. Advice on allergies and special diets.

Abbey Brook Cactus Nursery
Dept. CP, Bakewell Road
Matlock
Derbyshire DE4 2QJ

Supplies the cactus *Cereus Peruvianus*, which has been shown to absorb e/m radiation from VDUs and televisions.

British Holistic Medical Association
179 Gloucester Place
London NW1 6DX

British Society for Nutritional Medicine
PO Box 3AP
London W1A 3AP

College of Health
18 Victoria Park Square
London E2 9PF

Society for Environmental Therapy
3 Atherton Street
Ipswich, Suffolk IP4 2LD

McCarrison Society
24 Paddington St
London W1M 4DR

The Institute for the Study of Drug Dependence
1–4 Hatton Place
Hatton Garden
London EC1N 8ND

British Acupuncture Association
34 Alderney Street
London SW1V 4EU

National Institute of Medical Herbalists
PO Box 3
Winchester
Hants SO22 6RB

British School of Osteopathy (Mr Stephen Sandler DO MRO)
1–4 Suffolk Street
London SW1Y 4HG

Northern Natural Therapies
41 Teesway, Neasham
Darlington DL2 1QT

Pre-Menstrual Tension Advisory Service
PO Box 268
Hove, Sussex BN3 1RW

Counselling for *Candida* and Cystitis
Phone Angela Kilmartin (0171) 249 8664

British Society of Medical and Dental Hypnosis
42 Links Road
Ashtead
Surrey

Society of Teachers of the Alexander Technique
10 London House
266 Fulham Road
London SW10 9EL

Federation of Aromatherapists
46 Dalkeith Road
London SE21

Wholefood/Organically Grown Produce
24 Paddington Street
London W1M 4DR

Life Tool Holdings Ltd
Meridian House
Roe Street
Congleton
Cheshire CW12 1PG
(01260) 282000
Fax (01260) 282001

This firm has two new electronic medical machines. They work
with two ear clips at the press of a button. One reduces anxiety,
improves concentration, lifts depression and aids sleep (Alpha-Stim
SCS); the other does the same and also treats pain via probes
(Alpha-Stim 100). For £4.95 you can try the Alpha-Stim SCS for a
month without obligation to buy. It is a safe and effective treatment.

If you write to any of the above addresses please include an SAE.

Australia

Allergy Association
PO Box 298
Ringwood
Victoria 3134

Australian Institute of Health
Bennett House
Hospital Point
Acton
ACT 2601

Dept of Community Services and Health
Suite 60 MG
Parliament House
Canberra
ACT 2600

Women's Health Advisory Service
PO Box 1096
Bankstown
NSW 2200

USA

National Health Information Center
PO Box 1133
Washington DC

Women's Health Advisory Service
PO Box 31000
Phoenix
AZ 85046

Aeron Life Cycles Laboratory
1933 Davis Street
Suite 310
San Leandro
CA 94577
1-800-631-7900

The Nutritional Suppliers mentioned are willing to mail to America
or many of the same or similar products can be obtained from:

Interplexus Inc
6620 So 192nd Place
J-105 Kent
WA 98032

Further Reading

Allergy Connection, The, Barbara Paterson, (Thorsons, 1985).

Allergy Problem, The, Vicky Rippere, (Thorsons, 1983).

The Best is Yet To Come, Joseph Corvo, (Bedford Books, 1982).
    Available from PO Box 84, Croydon, Surrey, CR9 8BS.

British Medical Association Guide to Medicine and Drugs, The,
    (for prescription and over the counter medications), (Dorling
    Kindersley, 1989).

Candida Albicans: Could Yeast Be Your Problem, Leon Chaitow,
    (Thorsons, 1985).

Candida Albicans: Over 100 yeast-free and sugar-free recipes, Shirley
    Trickett, (Thorsons, 1995).

Cleansing the Colon, Brian Wright, available from New Nutrition,
    (see Useful Addresses).

Coming off Tranquillizers, Sleeping Pills and Antidepressants, Shirley
    Trickett, (Thorsons, 1986; 1998).

Coping with Anxiety and Depression, Shirley Trickett, (Sheldon
    Press, 1989).

Coping with Candida: Are Yeast Infections Draining Your Energy?,
    Shirley Trickett, (Sheldon Press, 1992).

Coping Successfully with Your Irritable Bowel, Rosemary Nicol, (Sheldon Press, 1989).

Coping Successfully with Panic Attacks, Shirley Trickett, (Sheldon Press, 1992; 5th impression 1998).

Daylight Robbery – The Importance of Sunlight to Health, (Arrow, 1998; available from Nutrition Associates).

Electropollution, Roger Coghill, (Thorsons, 1990).

Food Allergy and Intolerance, Jonathan Brostoff and Linda Gamlin, (Bloomsbury, 1989).

Food Combining for Health, Doris Grant and Jean Joice, (Thorsons, 1984).

Fully Human Fully Alive, John Powell, (Argus, 1976).

100% Health, Patrick Holford, (Piatkus, 1998).

Missing Diagnosis, The, C. Orion Truss, M.D. available from PO Box 25408, Birmingham AL 35226 USA.

More Self Help for Your Nerves and *The Latest Help for Your Nerves*, both by Claire Weekes, (Angus and Robertson, 1984, 1990).

Not All in the Mind, Richard Mackarness, (Pan, 1977).

Nutritional Medicine, Stephen Davies and Alan Stewart, (Bloomsbury, 1989).

Perhaps It's An Allergy, Ellen Rothera, (Foulsham, 1988).

The Practical Guide to Candida – Including Directory of UK Practitioners Who Treat Candida, Jane McWirter (Green Library, 1997; available from: 0171 385 0012).

Raw Energy, Leslie and Susannah Kenton, (Century Arrow, 1984).

Unconditional Love, John Powell, (Argus, 1979).

Wright Diet, The, Celia Wright, (Grafton, 1989).

Yeast Connection, The, William G. Crook M.D., (Biosocial Publications Europe).

References

'The Irritable Bowel Syndrome', *The Nursing Times*, vol. 83, Nov 1987, p. 51.

'The Irritable Bowel Syndrome: A Disease or a Response?' *Journal of the Royal Society of Medicine*, vol. 80, April 1987, p. 219.

'Hyperventilation and the Irritable Bowel Syndrome', *Lancet*, 25 Jan 1986, p. 221.

'Affective Illness and Zinc Deficiency', *Lancet*, 16 March 1985.

'Caffeine and Health', *British Medical Journal*, vol. 295, No. 6609, 21 Nov 1987, p. 1293.

Food Allergy and Intolerance, Jonathan Brostoff and Linda Gamlin, (Bloomsbury, 1989).

'Benzodiazepine Withdrawal, An Unfinished Story', *British Medical Journal*, vol. 288, 14 April 1984.

'Benzodiazepine Withdrawal Outcome in 50 patients', *British Journal of Addiction*, 82, 1987, pp. 665–671.

'Benzodiazepine Withdrawal: A review of the Evidence', *Journal of Clinical Psychiatry*, 49:10, October 1988.

'Addiction to Tranylcypromine', *British Medical Journal*, vol. 283, 1 August 1981.

'Effects of Physical Training on Mood', *J. Clin. Psychol.*, 32: 385, 1986.

'Anxiety Reduction Using Physical Exertion and Positive Images', Richard Driscoll, University of Colorado, *The Psychological Record* 26, 1976, pp. 87–94.

'Mood Alteration with Swimming', *Psychosom. Med.*, 45, 1983, pp. 425–433.

'Therapeutic Effects of Bright Light in Depressed Patients', Daniel F. Kripke, (Dept. Psychology, University of California, San Diego).

'Seasonal Variations in Affective Disorders', in Wohr and Goodwin (eds), *Circadian Rhythms in Psychiatry*, vol. 2, pp. 185–201 (Boxwood Press, Pacific Grove, Calif.).

Day Light Robbery, Damien Downing, (Arrow, 1988).

'Invasive Candidiasis following Cimetidine Therapy', *American Journal of Gastroenterology*, 1988 Jan 83 (1) 102–3.

'Candida Infections: An Overview', *CRC Critical Reviews in Microbiology*, vol. 15, 1.

'Urinary Tract Candiosis', *The Lancet*, 29 October 1988, pp. 1000–1.

'The Role of Candida Albicans in Human Illness', *Journal of Orthomolecular Psychiatry*, vol. 10, No. 4, 1981, pp. 228–38.

Electromagnetism and Life, Robert O. Becker and Andrew A. Marino, (State University of New York Press, Albany, New York, 1982), p. 211.

'The Effects of Therapeutic Touch on Anxiety Levels of Hospitalized Patients', Patricia Heidt, *Nursing Research*, 4 Feb 1980.

'Therapeutic Touch: A Facilitator of Pain Relief', Boguslawski, *Topics in Clinical Nursing*, vol. 2, No. 1, April 1980, pp. 27–39.

Index

glycaemic 118–19
high-fibre 93
low blood sugar 115–18
ME 86
prescribed drugs 94
smoking 42, 45
stomach 32, 35–6
ulcers 98
digestive system 9–11, 50, 54, 58
aromatherapy 207
Candida Albicans 73, 75
exercises 200–4
intolerances 88
low blood sugar 113
negative emotions 103
nervous system 66
stomach 33–4
diverticulitis 51, 193
Downing, Dr Damien 209
drugs 92–9, 152

edible intake 191
electromagnetic fields 148–51
emotions 6, 48, 103–6, 167, 175
enemas 15, 18
energy 152
enzymes 33–4, 50, 57
epilepsy 58
Epsom salts 58, 59
essential fatty acids (EFA) 28, 30–1, 164–5
essential oils 91, 205–9
Europe 84
evening primrose oil 30–1, 164–5
exercise 13, 15, 140–3
breathing 111–12
Candida Albicans 79, 83
colon 26
electrical fields 149
intolerances 90
lack 167
nervous system 68
poisons 43
relaxation 121

familial history 115
fat 48, 55, 116
fear 62–5, 109–11
Fitzgerald, Dr William 196
flatulence 18–23, 182–3
flax oil 30–1
folic acid 157
food combining 54, 60

food rotation 90
foot baths 58–9
Frankish, D. 87
Franklin, Mike 86
free radicals 159–60
fresh air 145–7, 166, 186
fruit 13–14, 42, 53
bowel 56–7, 59–60
Candida Albicans 78, 80
low blood sugar 116, 117
frustration 105
Fulder, Stephen 78
fungal infections 35, 72, 76, 99

Gaby, Alan 70
Galen 189
Gamlin, Linda 90
garlic 78–9, 83–4, 92, 116
Gillanders, Ann 198
Glucosamine 27
glycaemic diet 118–19
goat's milk 56, 59
Graham, Judy 165
Grant, Doris 54
Graphites 185
grief 104–5
guided imagery 122–5
guilt 106
gullet 9
gut flora 6, 17–18, 25, 37, 68, 86

haemorrhoids 16, 17
Hammond, Christopher 182
hangovers 47
head muscles 127–33
headaches 39, 40, 51–2, 59
colonic irrigation 193
diet 57
hyperventilation 108
intolerances 89
positive ions 145
prescribed drugs 98
relaxation 121
tension 103
Heidelberg Gastrogram Test 37
Herxheimer reaction 81
Hibbert, Dr 109–10
Higher Nature 27, 31, 71
Hippocrates 189
Homoeopathic Hospital, London 86
homoeopathy 22, 39, 181–6
hormones 70–1, 75, 119